NEW APPROACHES
TO
THEORY DEVELOPMENT

NEW APPROACHES TO THEORY DEVELOPMENT

Patricia Moccia, Editor

Pub. No. 15-1992

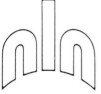

National League for Nursing • New York

Manufactured in the United States of America.

PREFACE

Martha E. Rogers has postulated that human development proceeds in wave patterns that are characterized by an ever-increasing frequency and complexity.[1] Theory development in nursing certainly supports this generalization. The number of studies and discussions on theory development in the nursing literature has proliferated in the ten years since *Theory Development: What? Why? How?* was first published by the National League for Nursing in 1975. In the last two years, at least four major texts on theory development or theoretical thinking in nursing have been published; before that, there was only one. There are now several collections of the works of the various theorists, when for years there was only the Riehl and Roy classic, and each of the theorists now has at least one text explicating her conceptual models. Finally, if the number of brochures that cross my desk is at all an accurate indicator, there has been an

---

1. M. E. Rogers, "Nursing: A Science of Unitary Man," in J. P. Riehl and C. Roy, eds., *Conceptual Models for Nursing Practice*, 2d ed. (New York: Appleton-Century-Crofts, 1980), p. 333.

v

almost exponential increase in the number of conferences, on-going work groups, research days, and so forth that address various aspects of the topic.

The nature and depth of the discussions have also changed dramatically in the last ten years. Where once nursing was on the defensive about why it should be concerned with theory de-velopment, the profession has moved far past that debate and is now vigorously engaged in fine-tuning the "what." The earlier questions about the appropriate areas of concern for nursing theory development have narrowed and become focused as a result of intensive investigations over the years concerning the meaning and characteristics of health, nursing, human phenom-ena, the environment, and the relationships among these four concepts, acknowledged as common to all nursing conceptual models.

Rogers has further postulated that this increasing complex-ity is incessantly innovative; again, theory development in nurs-ing demonstrates the principle. Discussions of the "how" of theory development initially entailed pragmatic requests for a recipe or formula. Today, the earlier question has developed into the debate about which methodologies are both appropriate and ade-quate for researching nursing's concerns. In turn, the contem-porary discussion has led us to reexamine the nature of nursing science and the interactive relationships it shares with various philosophies of science. The individual essays in this book fur-ther this discussion.

It has taken a certain amount of daring for the nursing profession, individual nurses, and these particular authors to engage in theory development activities. Each of us has some familarity with the radical implications of nurses' conceptual-izing and the threat that such activity seems to pose to the social order: We have only to remember nursing's struggles with in-stitutions, other professions, and the legal system to be "allowed" to make the jump from describing behavior to naming it. How many times have all of us written "patient appears to be sleep-ing" when we knew without a doubt that he or she was doing just that?

In a very real way, the works in this book demonstrate the complex and innovative process of theory development. The au-thors are courageous pioneers, each in her own way pushing back the frontiers of nursing science as she leads the way in areas that were once considered on the fringes of nursing scholarship but have since achieved legitimacy. Meleis, for example, has redirected the focus and emphasis of some of our scholarly investigations to domain concepts and questions; Quinn presents us with her work on therapeutic touch, one of the very few studies in the nursing literature that is an explicit testing of a nursing theory; and Hiestand has helped us rediscover our history and, in so doing, reconceptualize our present. Oiler is in the midst of arguing for phenomenology's respectability and acceptance in the world of nursing theory development, and Chopoorian and I have just begun the same journey in our respective discussions on the concept of environment and the relationship between theory and practice.

Each of the essays here, which was created especially for this volume, was written to present new answers to the questions of "why?" "what?" and "how?" None is presented as a final or definitive answer. But all will challenge you to approach our daily world of nursing in different and complex ways, to conceptualize anew, to dare to think, and, in so doing, to become engaged in theory development in nursing.

Patricia Moccia

ACKNOWLEDGMENTS

It almost goes without saying that this work is indebted to all those who have thought, spoken, and written about theory development in nursing over the years. But it owes its uniqueness to the willingness of the contributors to devote their time and studied thoughtfulness to this collection. All of the authors had added significantly to the science of nursing before they wrote the essays that appear in this book, and I refer the reader to their other works. As an editor, I appreciate their professionalism in this particular project; as a nurse, I respectfully appreciate their larger contributions.

P. M.

CONTENTS

Part I   *General Discussion*   *1*

Chapter 1   Theory Development and Domain Concepts
            Afaf Ibrahim Meleis, PhD, FAAN   *3*
Chapter 2   The Theory–Practice Dialectic
            Patricia Moccia, PhD, RN   *23*
Chapter 3   Reconceptualizing the Environment
            Teresa J. Chopoorian, EdD, RN   *39*

Part II   *Methodologies*   *55*

Chapter 4   Quantitative Methods: Descriptive and
            Experimental   *Janet F. Quinn, PhD, RN*   *57*
Chapter 5   Qualitative Methods: Phenomenology
            Carolyn J. Oiler, EdD, RN   *75*
Chapter 6   Conceptualizing Historical Research
            Wanda C. Hiestand, EdD, RN   *105*

Bibliography   *119*

Part I

General Discussion

1

THEORY DEVELOPMENT AND DOMAIN CONCEPTS

Afaf Ibrahim Meleis, PhD, FAAN
Professor, Department of Mental Health and Community Nursing
School of Nursing
University of California, San Francisco
San Francisco, California

INTRODUCTION

Members of some of the sciences from which nursing derives some of its knowledge have been involved in controversial ontological and epistemological debates whose aim is to replace an established set of ontological beliefs or mainstream epistemology with another set of assumptions and a methodology that is more congruent with the goals of the discipline. These sciences range from such well-established ones as physics to those that are still vying for scientific recognition, such as sociology and psychology. The methodological debates are subsequent to substantive debates, therefore allowing for cumulative knowledge development within the disciplines. While the knowledge being developed may have been limited to the existing ontology and epistemology of the field and thus may represent a biased view, it is the very

The author acknowledges the help of critical dialogues with doctoral and post-doctoral students in 1984–85 theory seminars (Nursing 202 A-B-C) in refining the ideas contained in this chapter.

nature of the disciplines' questions and propositions that has prompted the subsequent debates.

The discipline of nursing has followed a unique route in its knowledge development, which proceeded from debates about the structure of its knowledge rather than the substance of its content. Its debates ranged from whether there is a nursing theory or not to whether the methodological goals should be positivistic demons or phenomenological angels. Other debates included whether the discipline should use quantitative or qualitative research, Cartesian or hermeneutic science, basic or applied science, or feminist or traditional (masculine) methodology. Although these debates may be healthy, they might serve to divert the scientific community's energy from its primary task of developing knowledge related to the discipline's central questions.

My proposal here is not to halt all epistemological and ontological debates; I would suggest, however, that if these debates were focused on domain concepts and questions, they would offer a constructive potential to the development of nursing knowledge. The difference is more in the degree of emphasis and in the goals of the debates. A debate that is focused on whether phenomenology or hermeneutics is the more congruent methodology for the development of nursing knowledge would be more constructive if it focused on one of the domain questions in nursing as well. For example, a research program about the patterns of coping with transitions between health and illness and the most effective nursing therapeutics could be pursued using different ontological beliefs and methodological approaches.

Domain questions evolve from clinical practice and from the emerging domain assumptions and concepts. Debates on domain definitions could help bring about a more cumulative, integrative, and substantive future for the profession. The purpose of this chapter is to articulate some beginning definitions for domain concepts that reflect the major ontological beliefs of the discipline that have evolved from its shared oral history and its theorists. I offer these domain concepts so that clinicians can debate them, scientists can challenge them, theoreticians can tease out their inconsistencies, and all can further analyze them. The definitions also benefit from acknowledgment of the centrality of experience and perceptions in the development of nursing knowledge and the synthesis between several seemingly paradoxical principles.

The parallels between some of these principles and principles found in feminist theories are also briefly discussed. Although feminist methodologies have been propagated in other disciplines and differences between nonfeminist and feminist science have been demonstrated (such as in psychology), some of these principles have been an integral part of nursing practice but may have been ignored by nursing science in the past.

THE NURSING DOMAIN

The dimensions of a domain are conceptualized as follows:

1. A set of general and specific assumptions that are uniquely interrelated and upon which research, practice, theory, and education are based.
2. Some specific concepts and subconcepts that are derivable from the central concepts. General agreement on these concepts and their conceptual definitions should be apparent in the discipline's literature.
3. Identified major problem areas of the field which could make up the canons for significant propositions. The problem areas are based on the domain concepts and assumptions.
4. Identified major units of analysis or ongoing discussion about major and minor units of analysis.
5. A set of major research questions.
6. A set of agreed-upon methodologies.
7. Methodologies congruent with domain assumptions.
8. An openness in the domain to allow for continuity of discovery and development.

Central concepts in nursing have been identified through a review of nursing curricula[1] and through analysis of nursing theories.[2] A review and analysis of major assumptions related to these concepts and definitions within each of the nursing theories will help in pointing out congruencies and incongruencies and may therefore lead to identification of shared domain assumptions. Major domain assumptions as seen by nurse theorists are presented below. When theorists are not identified, it indicates my perception that the assumption is a shared view in nursing. Assumptions related to human responses, health and illness, the nursing client, the environment, interactions, and nursing therapeutics are presented, followed by major theorists' definitions of the human being, health, the environment, interactions, the nursing process, and nursing therapeutics.

ASSUMPTIONS

Human Responses

1. Human responses tend to be repetitive, orderly, organizable, predictable, and unified (Johnson; Levine; Rogers; Roy).
2. Human responses to health, actual health problems, or potential health problems are reflective of mind–body integration, and their problems as such are integrated (Johnson; Levine; Rogers).
3. Distress is the result of inability to cope with one's own needs (Orlando).

Health and Illness

1. Health and illness are inevitable conditions.
2. The illness experience exists as experienced and perceived by a person and caregivers (King; Paterson and Zderad; Rogers; Travelbee).
3. Illness experiences are self-actualizing if nurses and patients find meanings in them (Paterson and Zderad; Travelbee).
4. Health and well-being are both the rights and the responsibilities of individuals.

The Nursing Client

1. Nursing is concerned with the life processes of a human being (Donaldson and Crowley; Rogers).
2. Nurses are concerned with the needs of people related to health and illness (Henderson; Orem; Orlando; Wiedenbach).
3. Nursing is concerned with a unitary person, with a whole person (Paterson and Zderad; Rogers).
4. There is pattern, order, and organization in the wholeness of the unitary person (Johnson; Rogers; Wiedenbach).
5. Patients are unique and individual in their responses (Orlando; Travelbee; Wiedenbach).
6. Human beings attach meanings to situations and actions that may or may not be apparent to others (Orlando; Paterson and Zderad; Travelbee).
7. Energy can be mobilized to enhance healing (Krieger, Levine, Rogers).

8. Nursing clients are biopsychosociocultural spiritual beings (Johnson; Roy).
9. Individuals are continuously in interaction with their environments (King; Rogers; Roy).

Environment

1. It is assumed that nursing deals with people and their environments (Nightingale; Rogers).
2. It is assumed that environments influence individuals' responses and vice versa (Johnson; Nightingale; Rogers).

Interactions

1. Relationships between the nurse and patient are the essence of nursing and are established when each perceives the other's uniqueness (Travelbee; Paterson and Zderad).
2. The nurse–patient situation is dynamic; actions and reactions are influenced by both nurse and patient (King).

Nursing Therapeutics

1. Nursing acts influence the quality of a person's living and dying (Orlando; Travelbee).
2. Patients may need help in communicating needs, perceptions, thoughts, or feelings (Orlando).
3. Nursing actions are designed to bring about some positive consequence (ANA Social Policy Statement).
4. It is the responsibility of health care givers to inform individuals of all aspects of their care to help them make informed decisions (King).
5. Patients have the right to understand and participate in their own care, obtain information, and participate in decisions that may influence their own lives (King; Paterson and Zderad).
6. The dignity and integrity of human beings should be preserved in health and illness (Paterson and Zderad; Roy; Travelbee; WHO).

DEFINITIONS

The Human Being as a Nursing Client

1. A biopsychosocial being as a behavioral system threatened by loss of order, predictability, or stability because of illness or potential illness. "All patterned, repetitive, purposeful ways of behaving that characterize each man's life are considered to comprise his behavioral system."[3:209]

2. A person, family, group, or community, a biopsychosocial adaptive system with two processor subsystems that
   are mechanisms for adapting or coping with the regu-
   lator and the cognator. The system has four affectors of
   adaptation, or adaptive modes: physiological needs, self-
   concept, role function, and interdependence.[4:43] A holistic adaptive system.[5:36]

3. "An irreducible, four-dimensional, negentropic energy
   field identified by pattern-manifesting characteristics
   that are different from those of the parts and which
   cannot be predicted from knowledge of the parts."[6] This
   constitutes the man–environment relationship.[7:127] The
   unitary human being develops through three principles:
   helicy, resonancy, and complementarity.

4. A unique, total, open system with perception, self, body
   image, time, space, growth, and development throughout the life span, and with experiences of changes in
   structure and function of body influencing perception of
   self.[8:19–20] The person as an open system exhibits perme-
   able boundaries permitting an exchange of matter, energy, and information.[8:69]

5. A developmental human being who is under medical
   care and who cannot deal with his or her needs or who
   cannot carry out medical treatment alone.[9]

6. A human being who requests assistance knowing that
   the other can give assistance in solving health problems.
   A human being is always in the process of becoming.[10,11]

7. A person who is under the care of some member of the
   health care establishment, who is in a vulnerable position, and who has a perceived need for help.[12]

8. A total, whole person, a system of systems in a state of
   dissynchronization and in need of assistance to conserve
   energy and structural, personal, and social integrity.[13,14]
   A person is always changing, because of continual interaction with the environment, and is constantly striving to maintain integration.

9. A human being with health-related or health-derived
   limitations rendering him incapable of continuous self-
   care when self-care requisites exceed self-care capability.[15]

Health

1. Efficient and effective functioning of the system. Bal-
   ance and stability of the behavioral system.[3]

2. A state of adaptation that is manifested in free energy

to deal with other stimuli. A process of promoting integrity.[5:39]

3. "Characteristics and behaviors emerging out of the mutual, simultaneous interaction of the human and environmental fields."[16] Greater developmental coherence that evolves from human–environment energy fields that are novel, emerging, and diverse in pattern and organization.

4. A dynamic life experience of a human being, which implies continuous adjustment to stressors in the internal and external environment through optimum use of one's resonances to achieve potential for daily living.[8:5,17:186]

5. Sense of adequacy or well-being, fulfilled needs, sense of comfort.[9:9]

6. Greater well-being.[10:12]

7. A state of complete physical, mental, and social well-being, not merely the absence of disease or infirmity. The enjoyment of the highest attainable standards of health is one of the fundamental rights of every human being without distinction of race, religion, or political, economic, or social condition.[11,18]

8. Patterns of adaptive change.[19:2452] Retention of integrity and wholeness.

9. Structural or functional wholeness, soundness, and integrity.[15:118–19]

Environment

1. All conditions, circumstances, and influences, internal and external, that may affect the development and behavior of persons and groups. The focal, contextual, and residual stimuli that influence individuals' responses.[5:39]

2. An irreducible four-dimensional negentropic energy field, identified by patterns and manifesting characteristics different from those of the parts and encompassing any given human field.[6:222]

3. The internal environment of human beings transforms energy to enable them to adjust to continuous external environment changes.[8:5] External environment is a formal and informal organization.

4. The objective world of people and things and the subjective meaning of people and things.[10]

5. A conglomeration of objects, policies, setting, atmosphere, time, humans, and happenings past, current, or anticipated that is dynamic, unpredictable, exhilarating, baffling, and disruptive.[20:1061]

6. A setting, a background, and the dynamic exchange that involves both the individual organism and the setting and background. It is perceptual (one's own interpretation), operational (e.g., virus) and conceptual (culture).[13:12,14:94]

Interactions

1. "A process of perception and communication between person and environment and between person and person, represented by verbal and nonverbal behaviors that are goal oriented."[8:145]
2. The human dialogue is the essence of nursing: nursing is interaction. The nurse–patient experience is an intersubjective transaction with empathy.[10]
3. An experience between an individual in need of the services of a nurse, and a nurse, for the purpose of meeting the needs of the patient.[11]
4. The deliberate use of nurses' perceptions, thoughts, feelings, and actions.[12]
5. Automatic activities such as perception by the five senses, thoughts, feelings, and actions. Disciplined and professional activities, which are automatic activities plus matching of verbal and nonverbal responses, validation of perceptions and responses, and matching of thoughts and feelings with action.[21:25–32]
6. Interaction is dependent on perceptual systems of two individuals.[22:97]

Nursing Process

1. A "particular format" used in nursing that utilizes the problem-solving approach. It comprises the six steps of assessment of behaviors, assessment of influencing factors, nursing diagnosis, goal setting, intervention, and evaluation.[5:42–62]
2. Purposeful interaction with clients to share information, set mutual goals, participate in decisions about goals and means, and implement plans and evaluation.[8]
3. The interaction between the patient's behaviors, the nurse's reactions, and the nurse's actions for the purpose of patient benefits.[9:36]
4. "Deliberate, responsible, conscious, aware, nonjudgmental existence of the nurse in the nursing situation, followed by disciplined, authentic reflections and description"[10:7–8] based on continuous assessment and development of the patient's human potential for responsible choosing between alternatives.[10]

5. A "disciplined intellectual approach," a logical method of approaching nursing problems to ascertain needs, validate inferences, decide who should meet needs, plan course of action, and validate that course.[11]

6. Deliberative process undertaken to identify needs for help and interferences with ability to cope. Use of observation, understanding, and clarification of meaning of cues, determination of causes of discomfort, of whether patient is able to meet own needs. Includes ministration of help, validation, and evaluation.[12:56–57]

7. Assessment, diagnosis, and intervention, using steps of the scientific method with emphasis on observation.[13:23–29]

8. A system to determine need for care, plan for care, and implementation of care.[15]

Nursing Therapeutics

1. Regulate and control by providing protection, nurturance, or stimulation to subsystems and by external mechanisms restricting, defending, inhibiting, or facilitating these subsystems.[3,23]

2. Traditional techniques such as comfort measures, or entirely new activities that have not as yet been discovered, all with the goal of promoting adaptation.[4:47–48]

3. Repatterning of human and environment energy fields for more effective fulfillment of life's capabilities.[7:127]

4. Transactions that inform and share in the setting of mutual goals. Participation in decisions about goals and the means to achieve them. Goal-oriented nursing record.[17:183–6]

5. Whatever help the patient may require for his needs to be met.[9:5] Includes suggesting, directing, explaining, informing, requesting, questioning, handling the body of the patient. Includes both automatic activities and deliberative activities.

6. A human dialogue that involves being and doing, nurturing, well-being or greater well-being, nurturance and comfort by experiencing, reflecting, and conceptualizing an existential existence. Nurses offer alternatives and support choices.[10]

7. Therapeutic use of self in a disciplined and intellectual approach to patient problems to enable them to cope with the stress of illness and suffering. Helping patients find meaning in their experiences.[24:10] Detailed methods are provided by Travelbee[24] and Meleis.[25:159]

8. Deliberate action (help) that is nurse- or patient-

directed, or both, to restore and extend a patient's ability to cope with the demands implicit in his or her situation and to function capably (through giving advice, information, referral, ministry, etc.).[12]

9. Creating an atmosphere in which healing can occur; therefore, the target is the environment. Conserve patient resonances, alter the environment to fit the resonances. Act as the patient's perceptual system.[19,26]

10. Deliberate, systematic, and purposeful action. Totally compensatory, partly compensatory, or educative supportive care in universal, developmental, and health deviation self-care deficits.[15:55-85]

HUMAN PHENOMENA: NECESSARY CONDITIONS

Nursing phenomena are human phenomena. They represent the experiences of nurses and clients; both are human beings and participants in the health care system. As such, certain factors guide their further development; two of these that are also themes in the domain assumptions are experience and perception. The synthesis between several paradoxes is also a condition for this development: the paradoxes of particularism and holism, uniqueness and generalization. Each of these conditions is discussed below.

THEMES

Experience. *Experience* in this case denotes clinical experience, including that of nurses and that of patients. Nurses have gone about doing the business of nursing care all over the world. Some have been aware of the use of theories in their practices, others may have used theory without being aware of it, and still others have claimed they relied on their own experiences and those of others in delivering nursing care. There are those who vehemently continue to argue that they have not used theory and do not need nursing theory to perform all actions inherent in nursing practice. In spite of these variations in determination of the use of theory, nurses agree that nursing care is different from other forms of health care and that a nurse's view of the patient, the situation, and the intervention may differ from that of other health professionals in emphasis, content, or goals. Other health professionals may argue about the significance of these differences, but on the whole all agree that health care clients are better off receiving the multiplicity of care given by the various health professionals.

All health professionals would agree that one of the most significant sources of theories in their respective disciplines lies in the sphere of health care. Nursing is no exception. Nursing practice is the arena from which we describe phenomena and discover relationships between phenomena, as well as invent potential relationships between phenomena. Invention is particularly helpful when considering clinical therapeutics in the process of development. These, then, represent the soil from which theories can grow. Theories help to articulate pragmatic research questions, the answers to which lend support to early hunches or shed new light on them by leading to further questions.

The experience of nurses in providing nursing care for clients was the impetus for one of the first theoretical formulations in nursing.[27] Nursing as it is is as significant as nursing as it should be in the development of theoretical and research questions. I have become more convinced than ever that this is so as I undertake more international nursing and listen to colleagues' frustrations about nursing theories because of their lack of utility in their own countries. The most significant reasons for that lack of utility is the actual nursing role in a country that precludes direct patient care. My advice to them, and to all of us, is to conceptualize nursing in terms of the goals of nursing in that particular country, the object and subject of care given, the actions given, and the structure within which the care is given. What better way to do that than by relying on nurses' experiences?

The significance of experience in developing theories becomes even more apparent when viewed as a significant principle in feminist methodology. In advocating feminist methodology, sociologists and psychologists have supported clinical experience as a source for the development of theory and for making sense out of research data.[28] Nursing has a built-in mechanism for observation of phenomena within the naturalistic environment of care.

Feminist methodology also supports the importance of discussions between subjects and researchers or theoreticians.[28] It treats subjects as participants and relies on their verifications of an emerging explanation and its meaning. Nurse clinicians have observed clinical phenomena and discussed their meaning with clients. They have also developed conceptual relationships based on theories. Many of these conceptualizations have remained on an individual basis and have not been adequately valued or shared.

Perceptions. Closely tied with experience is the principle of perception. Nurses observe, touch, smell, think, and feel patients' behaviors, needs, and problems. Then they attribute a meaning to what was manifested. The combination of all these is perception. During this process, nurses bounce their perceptions off on patients and modify these perceptions with those of the patients, who also have their own perceptions of their behaviors, needs, and problems. Nurses then plan their actions.

Perceptions are a significant dimension in defining theory or research in nursing. The result of this shift from the received view (objective, sensory data, free of values) to the perceived view (a view that accepts values, subjectivity, intuition, history, tradition, and multiple realities) is a view that is more congruent with nursing and its focus on human phenomena.[25,29–31]

PARADOXES

Particularism and Holism. More and more, nursing literature is supporting a holistic view of nursing clients. Some of the theories that have been useful in providing explanations and understanding of client health behaviors have conceptualized clients and nursing therapeutics more from a particularistic view than a holistic view. A particularistic view tends to reduce human beings into subsystems of behavior (Johnson), adaptive modes (Roy), or self-care problems (Orem). Others have addressed human beings as a whole and admonished nursing to study their coordinated integrated responses (Rogers).

Patients who present problems have always been the focus of medical science and are what nursing is concerned with in many existing institutions. Therefore, by eliminating particularistic or problem-focused approaches from our theoretical literature, we may not be allowing the development of knowledge based on clinical practice, which is based on this particularism.

Particularism and holism are dimensions of each phase of the nursing process. In the assessment phase, a nurse with a particularistic approach may focus on the problem or a subsystem and manifestation of the problem. A holistic nurse would focus on the whole person, on how the problem may be influencing the patient's quality of life, the meaning of the problem, and the patient's perception of how the problem arose. A particularistic therapeutic would focus on caring for the immediate problem, while a holistic approach would include future prevention of the problem and, perhaps, a view of how the proposed nursing therapeutic may be used with other, similar problems.[32]

The limitations of our knowledge and methodologies, and the complexity and many dimensions of human phenomena, do not permit the adoption of one view to the exclusion of the others. Observing, theorizing about, and researching the affiliative subsystems of behavior or the role functions of certain clients in response to a life-threatening disease could provide us with necessary data that is significant to the care of these clients; it would also help us to consider clients' total integrated responses to the same conditions.

Uniqueness and Generalization. Theory and science presume the potential for generalization, yet one of the most significant assumptions in nursing is that it considers and respects the uniqueness of its clients. This seeming paradox has kept the scientists, the theoreticians, and the clinicians apart intellectually. Clinicians, having experienced the diversity of their clients, express a very strong and legitimate need to preserve that uniqueness. The empiricists and theoreticians, seeking the development of a nursing knowledge base, seek the development of generalizations. Because of that seeming paradox, clinicians' experiences and perceptions may have been slow in being communicated conceptually.

The challenge in dealing with human phenomena is in the ability to develop theories that meet the assumptions of both practice and science. It is possible to do that if the concept or the relationship under exploration is considered within the context of the human situation. That is, situational variables and contextual conditions must be delineated to depict the potential diversity in responses. An example of this is the ongoing research and theory work of the Mid-East SIHA project (Study of Immigrants' Health and Adjustment) at the University of California, San Francisco. As we conceptualize the experience of immigration, transition, and the consequences on health, therefore attempting to make some generalizations, we consider numerous contexts and situations. Some of these may be personal variables, such as education and occupation, while others are sociocultural, such as type of immigration and attitudes toward immigration in the mother country as well as in the host country.

The goals of the research program are to develop theories that describe the different probable scenarios. From a nursing perspective, the most important focus is on the human–environment interactions and the health of the individual and community; therefore, personal and cultural perceptions and experiences and the meaning of transition and health to the individual client would help to give a sense of individual variation. These perceptions, experiences, meanings, and principles synthesize the seemingly opposite views of uniqueness and generalization. They allow for many practice-oriented generalizations that could formulate the concepts and relationships in developing theories without abrogating the principle of human individuality and human uniqueness.

Genderless or Nonsexist Theories. As we consider these conditions, the influence of the feminist scientific process becomes apparent. It is a process that has been conceptualized to be more qualitative than quantitative[33] and is based on existential philosophies and phenomenological approaches. It considers women's experiences and their perceptions, treats subjects as participants, and looks at data analysis as meaningful only within a specific context. It influences the type of questions asked and the processes for developing answers. Nursing deals with human phenomena of both males and females. Though developments in women's studies may have appropriately and profoundly influenced nursing, perhaps what is emerging is a genderless approach to theory development.

ON DEFINING NURSING PHENOMENA

Nursing is a human science that deals with human and environmental responses or potential responses to health and illness situations. Its goals are to mobilize human and environmental resources to promote healing, maintain well-being, prevent illness, and promote health. As such, the domain of nursing encompasses the health and well-being of human beings who are in interaction with their environments, who may be undergoing or anticipating some kind of transition related to health and illness. Nurses use certain processes and a variety of clinical therapeutics to deal with these human and environmental responses.

It has been the intent of this chapter to identify the premises and principles that guide the definitions of central nursing phenomena in relationship to nursing practices and to delineate the conditions necessary for the study of such phenomena. A running theme of the chapter has been the influence of feminist theories on the development of knowledge in nursing and the influence of the recent interest in women's health on the development of understanding of human phenomena that are of interest to nursing.

SYNTHESIS OF ASSUMPTIONS AND DEFINITIONS

The synthesis of assumptions and definitions of nursing phenomena that has emerged from nursing theories, with the seeming incongruencies and paradoxes created by the realities of practice and the perceived canons of science, has helped in the development of working definitions for the central nursing phenomena. These definitions, seen below, show the potential uniqueness of individuals from both a particularistic and a holistic view of human beings. Each of the definitions should be used within the context of perceptions, experiences, and meanings as principles for further theory development.

Nursing Client. A nursing client is defined as a biopsychosocio-cultural being who is unable or at risk of being unable to care for the self. The nursing client is an open system, an adaptive being who is continually changing to accommodate to surrounding changes. The nursing client has some basic needs as well as some unique needs, some of which are not being met because of health or illness situations. The nursing client is in disequilibrium or at risk of being in disequilibrium. A human being may be sick or well and may or may not be a nursing client. He or she would not become a nursing client unless one of the above properties existed.

A nursing client may or may not be a client of other members of the health team, and, when cared for by other members, may be discharged from any one of the services independently of others, except for hospitalization. A patient who needs medical attention also needs nursing care. To adequately and effectively assess a client's situation, needs, and requirements for immediate and long-term care, a nurse utilizes a framework that she may be aware of but is usually unable to articulate.

Health. Health is defined as a sense of biopsychosocial well-being and coherence as perceived by a human being and others and as manifested in efficient and effective capabilities to function, cope, and adjust to life experiences. Health is also manifested in the ability to use internal and external resources in dealing with life experiences.

Environment. Environment includes the setting, the background, and the conditions that surround and encompass the nursing client or are anticipated to do so. Theories centering on the environment would describe properties, components, and dimensions of the environment that are healthy or that may help in maintaining or promoting health. Such theories would describe the environment that promotes the nursing client's self-care, adaptation, and effective interventions.

Interaction. According to *Webster's New Collegiate Dictionary*, interaction is "the interchange, exchange, and mutual reciprocal action or influence" of a human being with the environment or with the nurse. It is through interaction that perceptions may be explored and responses may be articulated as a dynamic process in which two or more human beings participate in an exchange or interchange and influence each other, or in a process in which a human being and the environment influence each other. It is a process in which sensing, communicating, intuiting, perceiving, validating, and empathizing may occur. The objective of interaction is to develop rapport, an understanding of the client and the nursing–client situation, and an assessment of the client's needs, to interpret and validate development of a shared meaning for the development of goals in health–illness situations. Interaction also encompasses the reciprocal influence of nursing clients and their environment (significant others, aggregate, society, organization). Finally, an interaction may be a clinical therapeutic.

Nursing Process. The nursing process is a tool for nursing practice; it is deliberate, systematic, and goal-oriented. It includes two major goals: assessment and choice of nursing therapeutics. Tools for the process are observation, intuition, reflection, writing, communication, assessment, and choice of alternative actions. It is continuous, flexible, and collaborative. It includes the nurse, client, significant others, family, and other team members.

Transition. Transition refers to the period in which a change is perceived by a person or others, as occurring in a person or in the environment. There are some commonalities that characterize a transition period: (1) disconnectedness from usual social network and social support systems, (2) temporary loss of familiar reference points or significant objects or subjects, (3) new needs that may arise or old ones not met in a familiar way, and (4) old sets of expectations no longer congruent with changing situations. A transition denotes a change in health status, in role relations, in expectations, or in abilities. Responses or potential responses to transition are within the domain of nursing.

Nursing Therapeutics. Nursing therapeutics include *all* nursing activities and actions deliberately designed to care for nursing clients and to assist in preserving energy for healing, mobilizing inner and outer resources to enhance coping with health and illness situations, and maintaining a sense of comfort and well-being. They include actions designed to promote and maintain health and health behavior.

CONCLUSION

Theories in nursing have evolved out of some shared and some diverse views of nursing and its goals. These views are useful in raising meaningful research questions that depend on the nature of the situation. No single theory by itself can answer all the practice questions. Each attempts to answer some of the questions, but the complexity of nursing, stemming from its contextuality, the nurse's concern with the patient as a whole, the patient's relationship with the environment, and nursing's goal of promoting well-being, does not make it feasible or useful to develop one grand theory to answer all questions related to nursing care of patients. Nursing deals with many varied dimensions, present and future: with the individual, the family, and aggregates; with a cell, a limb, and a whole. Therefore, understanding, explanations, and prescriptions are possible only when several different theories are used and when different theories are developed to answer the many central questions in nursing.

Several trends have affected the development of theoretical nursing: a shift from an interest in medical phenomena that was focused mainly on cure, illness, prescribed tasks, and the duality in relationships between the person delivering the care and the person receiving the care to an emphasis on care, environment, and the perception and meaning of the situation of all individuals. The shift has also been toward encouraging clients' active participation in their own health care and the collaboration of all those involved in the care. These appear to be conditions that have grown out of advances in feminist methodologies. Current definitions of nursing phenomena emerge from a synthesis of all these conditions as well as from the fine work that our pioneer nurses provided us. These definitions are the impetus for further theoretical developments within the discipline of nursing.

NOTES

1. H. Yura and G. Torres, "Today's Conceptual Frameworks within Baccalaureate Nursing Programs," in *Faculty Curriculum Development, Part III: Conceptual Framework—Its Meaning and Function* (New York: National League for Nursing, 1975).
2. J. H. Flaskerud and E. J. Halloran, "Areas of Agreement in Nursing Theory Development," *Advances in Nursing Science*, 3 (October 1980): 1–7.
3. D. E. Johnson, "The Behavioral System Model For Nursing," in J. P. Riehl and C. Roy, eds., *Conceptual Models for Nursing Practice* (New York: Appleton-Century-Crofts, 1980).
4. C. Roy and S. Roberts, *Theory Construction in Nursing: An Adaptation Model* (Englewood Cliffs, New Jersey: Prentice-Hall, 1981).
5. C. Roy, *Introduction to Nursing: An Adaptation Model*, 2d ed. (Englewood Cliffs, New Jersey: Prentice-Hall, 1984).
6. M. E. Rogers, "Science of Unitary Human Being: A Paradigm for Nursing," in I. W. Clements and F. B. Roberts, eds., *Family Health: A Theoretical Approach to Nursing Care* (New York: John Wiley & Sons, 1983).
7. M. E. Rogers, *An Introduction to the Theoretical Basis of Nursing* (Philadelphia: F. A. Davis, 1970).
8. I. M. King, *A Theory for Nursing: Systems, Concepts, Process* (New York: John Wiley & Sons, 1981).
9. I. Orlando, *The Dynamic Nurse–Patient Relationship* (New York: Putnam, 1961).
10. J. G. Paterson and L. T. Zderad, *Humanistic Nursing* (New York: John Wiley & Sons, 1976).
11. J. Travelbee, *Interpersonal Aspects of Nursing*, 2d ed. (Philadelphia: F. A. Davis, 1971).
12. E. Wiedenbach, "The Helping Art of Nursing," *American Journal of Nursing*, 63 (1963): 54–57.
13. M. E. Levine, *Introduction to Clinical Nursing*, 2d ed. (Philadelphia: F. A. Davis, 1973).

14. M. E. Levine, "The Science Is Spurious," *American Journal of Nursing*, 79 (1979): 1379–83.
15. D. M. Orem, *Nursing: Concepts of Practice*, 2d ed. (New York: McGraw-Hill, 1980).
16. M. E. Rogers, *The Science of Unitary Man* (New York: Media for Nursing video tapes, 1980).
17. I. M. King, "King's Theory of Nursing," in I. W. Clements and F. B. Roberts, eds., *Family Health: A Theoretical Approach to Nursing Care* (New York: John Wiley & Sons, 1983).
18. World Health Organization (WHO), *Declaration of Alma Ata*, International Conference of Primary Health Care, Alma Ata, September 1978.
19. M. Levine, "Adaptation and Assessment: A Rationale for Nursing Intervention," *American Journal of Nursing*, 66 (1966): 2450–54.
20. E. Wiedenbach, "Nurses' Wisdom in Nursing Theory," *American Journal of Nursing*, 70 (1970): 1057–62. .
21. I. Orlando, *The Discipline and Teaching of Nursing Process* (New York: Putnam, 1972).
22. M. Levine, "The Pursuit of Wholeness," *American Journal of Nursing*, 69 (1969): 93–98.
23. D. E. Johnson, "The Significance of Nursing Care," *American Journal of Nursing*, 61 (1961): 63–66.
24. J. Travelbee, *Interpersonal Aspects of Nursing* (Philadelphia: F. A. Davis, 1966).
25. A. I. Meleis, *Theoretical Nursing: Development and Progress* (Philadelphia: J. B. Lippincott, 1985).
26. M. Levine, "The Four Conservation Principles of Nursing," *Nursing Forum*, 6 (1967): 45–59.
27. F. Nightingale, *Notes on Nursing: What It Is and What It Is Not* (New York: Dover, 1969).
28. B. S. Wallston, "What Are the Questions in Psychology of Women? A Feminist Approach to Research," *Psychology of Women Quarterly*, 5 (1981): 597–617.
29. P. L. Munhall, "Nursing Philosophy and Nursing Research: In Apposition or Opposition," *Nursing Research*, 31 (1982): 175–77.
30. C. Oiler, "The Phenomenological Approach in Nursing Research," *Nursing Research*, 31 (1982): 178–181.
31. P. Winstead-Fry, "The Scientific Method and Its Impact on Holistic Health," *Advances in Nursing Science*, 2 (July 1980): 1–7.
32. S. H. Kim, *The Nature of Theoretical Thinking in Nursing* (Norwalk, Connecticut: Appleton-Century-Crofts, 1983).
33. K. I. MacPherson, "Feminist Methods: A New Paradigm for Nursing Research," *Advances in Nursing Science*, 5 (January 1983): 17–25.

2

THEORY DEVELOPMENT AND NURSING PRACTICE: A SYNOPSIS OF A STUDY OF THE THEORY–PRACTICE DIALECTIC

Patricia Moccia, PhD, RN
Associate Professor and Chair
Department of Nursing Education
Teachers College, Columbia University
New York, New York

INTRODUCTION

"I'm a doer, not a thinker." In a New York City mayoral campaign in the late 1970s, the doer-not-a-thinker candidate spent hundreds of thousands of dollars repeating this slogan to the voting population. The fact that he did not get elected is a reflection neither on his doing nor on his not thinking; nor is it an index of the desires of New Yorkers for the opposing candidate, whom we might assume was a thinker, not a doer. In order to understand the election results, we would need a fairly comprehensive analysis that included, at least, the positions of the other candidates in relation to the voters and to each other; the relationship of the election and its promises to the myriad of other experiences that New Yorkers were then living through and those they had lived through previously; and the relationship of that local contest to past, present, and future elections at the state and federal level. In short, the most thorough explanation of the election results would depend upon context for its completeness.

Centuries of philosophical debate became focused in that single election promise, as they had in various other contexts in other societies at other times. Who holds the more vital role in any society, the action person or the philosopher? Was it the knights and warriors who preserved the kingdom or the philosopher-king and his council? Was the war waged, won, and lost by the grunts on the line or by those diplomats and government leaders who decided the shape of the table for the peace talks and the conditions of the peace treaty? Was the championship basketball game decided by the skills of the players on the court or the locker-room strategies of the coach?

The broader philosophical question of the relationship between theory and practice takes various forms as it moves closer to nursing's concerns. Is nursing a science or an art? Is nursing theory applied to practice or developed from it? What are the differences between professional and technical nursing, and which is the "real" nursing? Who is the "real" nurse—the scholar or the clinician?

A premise of this chapter is that there is a dialectical relationship between nursing theory and nursing practice in which both share an ongoing series of interactions through which each defines itself and determines its nature in relation to the other; and that there is a similiar relationship between nursing theoreticians or scholars and nursing practitioners. The term *theory* is used in one of its broadest, most inexact interpretations—as a way of looking at and understanding the world—and includes the terms "conceptual systems," "conceptual models," "theoretical systems," "theoretical models," and "theories." This is not to imply any disregard or disrespect for the distinctions between the terms or the importance of knowing the differences, but merely to leave that discussion to other arenas and to focus on similarities rather than differences.

Theory, as defined by Kaplan, is

> the device for interpreting, criticizing and unifying established laws, modifying them to fit data unanticipated in their formulation, and guiding the enterprise of discovering new and more powerful generalizations. . . . Theory is in this respect properly contrasted with *practice*; and "theoria" is contemplation viewed as something distinct from action. It is crucial, however, that the contrast make sense only when referred to the context of the problemmatic situation in which we are taking thought. In an enlarged context, theorizing

may be a very practical activity indeed and contemplation may be another kind of action, neither passive nor disengaged.[1:295]

Rather than existing in opposition, nursing theory and nursing practice depend on each other for their ongoing development. Therefore, rather than struggling to choose between nursing theory and nursing practice as alternatives, nurses can approach the issue most productively by rephrasing the question to account for the internal relationship between the two. This paper addresses that new question: How can the inherent dialectical relationship between nursing theory and nursing practice be used to advance nursing science?

CONTEMPORARY FORMS OF A HISTORICAL QUESTION

During the early phases of nursing theory development (1950–1970), particular themes filled the literature with editorials and letters to the editors, position papers and reactions to position papers, scholarly essays, and their critiques. Certainly, the "What?" "Why?" and "How?" questions of that time have moved a lot closer to resolution. Although Conway has recently argued for greater specificity when discussing or researching the concept of "nursing,"[2] it continues to be included, along with "persons," "health," and "environment," in the four concepts central to the discipline's research and theory-building activities.[3,4] As Chinn and Jacobs discuss,[5:21] there is a general recognition within the profession that theory development provides nursing with the basis for professional autonomy, coherence of purpose, and professional communication. In addition, the profession has closed ranks around why we need nursing theory in the cause of presenting a united front against the direct and indirect attempts to encroach on our boundaries.[6]

But the how of theory development remains a perplexing problem for nursing scholarship as today's literature is marked by the debate on which method for nursing research is appropriate or adequate for nursing's concerns.[7–10] On one hand, the growing popularity of various qualitative methods has enriched nurse researchers' repertoires as a result of the recognition that the nature of the question or problem is one of the most significant factors in choosing how to study it.[11] On the other, however, there continues to be a certain degree of tension about where these problems are to be found[12] and who can best legitimize the questions asked.[13] The root of the ongoing discussion is whether the research question begins with practical problems, is resolved in theory, and then applied to the practice situation, or whether the question is both identified and resolved in theoretical discourse and practice and then adapts itself to the findings.

While many say they accept practice as the determining element,[14] there continue to be inconsistencies between proclamations and actions. The chances are slim, for instance, that a free-standing clinic will receive research funds rather than a university health center, or that a senior nurse clinician without a doctorate will be awarded grant monies without a doctorally prepared colleague, regardless of her expertise, being designated as the principal investigator. Still another example of the theory or practice debate is the ongoing heated controversy over the appropriate entry requirements for professional nursing practice, which in the extreme has been described as a choice between a "competent nurse" (the doer) and "another unspecialized dilettante" (the thinker).[15]

The intense debates over the differences between theories, conceptual systems, models, and frameworks no longer dominate the literature as they did in the earlier phases of nursing's theoretical evolutions, since a general consensus on the common and distinguishing characteristics of each of the terms has been reached. What do continue to be questioned, however, are the different criteria with which to evaluate the various models and systems. Ellis, for example, was concerned with evaluating a theory for its significance,[16] and Hardy for its adequacy.[17] Reflecting the early concerns of theorists, Duffey and Muhlenkamp ask the most general of questions,[18] while Stevens, at a later stage of nursing's theory development, presented a sophisticated means for internal and external judgements.[19:49-68] Most recently, Chinn and Jacobs,[5:130-45] Fawcett,[20] and Meleis[14] have each presented a set of criteria that reflect their concerns for nursing theories.

An obvious question that emerges from these examples is how to select the evaluation criteria. More specifically, which critique will reveal a theory or way of looking at the world that is potentially most relevant for practice? In light of nursing's historic and contemporary commitment to promoting, maintaining, and restoring people's health, the specific question becomes, "What theory or way of understanding reality has the most promising possibilities for the practitioner working with people to maximize their health potential?"

THE DIALECTICS OF THE THEORY–PRACTICE RELATIONSHIP

Any discussion of the dialectical relationship between theory and practice obviously begins with an understanding of the dialectic, which has alternately been described as a philosophy or world view, a method of inquiry, a method of exposition, an intellectual process of incorporating new information into already existing explanations of phenomena, and any one or combination of these.[21] Whichever of these definitions one uses, the dialectic develops from three basic assumptions: (1) what appears to be reality is only and always a part of a larger whole; (2) the nature of the whole and all its parts is continually and incessantly changing into its next developmental stage; and (3) the whole is known through the network of internal dialectical relationships that exist among its parts.[22] Therefore, the dialectical relationship between theory and practice and that between scholars and practitioners necessarily develop from the same assumptions. Since all defining characteristics of dialectical relationships will develop from and manifest these assumptions, they are a logical starting point for evaluating theory.

Nursing is not the only discipline concerned with the relationship between theory and practice, as any review of the literature will show. Dialecticians, especially, have spent considerable time studying the nature of the interaction between the two seemingly opposite ways of apprehending reality—either through theory or practice. The works of Georg Lukacs, Antonio Gramsci, and Jurgen Habermas are among some of the most prominent and influential discussions of the theory–practice dialectic, and the most central works of each of these individuals have been studied for their relevance to nursing theory development.[6]

Lukacs, Gramsci, and Habermas were philosophers and social scientists whose works, not surprisingly, do not directly address the concept of health. Nonetheless, their significance for nursing is easily inferred because of their concerns with the arguably parallel concept of "freedom," wherein people are considered free to the extent that they are aware, active participants (subjects) in their lives or in the making of their history.[6:83-85] It was argued that the actualization of this potential to be free would include those same activities that would allow the subject's health potential to be realized. Since these works are concerned with the ways in which certain theories or approaches to understanding reality either promote or restrict the growth and development of freedom (or health), the study was able to synthesize the list of additional measures for evaluating nursing theory that is outlined below.

EVALUATION: DOES THE THEORY SERVE THE PURPOSES OF THE PROFESSION?

It has become a matter of course that theories are to be evaluated according to certain internal and external criteria. In addition to measuring nursing's theoretical systems by specific standards in both these areas, nurses are now returning to a variation of the earlier question of "Why theory development?" With a specificity gained from dialogue over the last several years, nurses are developing ways to assess whether the values and assumptions of a theory match those of the profession and, if so, whether the theory's potential is to foster or to impede the goals of nursing practice. In other words, which theories or approaches to reality have the greatest potential to allow and enhance the development of a practice that, in turn, has the greatest potential to do the same for people's health? Or, will the theory serve the purposes of the profession?

It is at this point that the dialectical nature of the relationship between theory and practice becomes a significant factor in selecting evaluation criteria. Within a dialectical understanding of the world, theory and practice share a codetermining interaction through which each grows, develops, and changes. Since one can, therefore, match certain characteristics of theories with corollary characteristics in practice, an assessment of one can serve as a predictor of the other. The following have been extracted from the assumptions and contradictions of the dialectic and from attempts to apply them. They are presented as the minimal attributes for a theoretical approach that has a greater potential to promote rather than restrict the development of health. As part of a dialectical universe, the attributes are themselves dialectical; in other words, they develop in relation to each other and to the whole, as will be seen in the following discussion.

ASSUMPTIONS OF THE DIALECTIC

The first two criteria are condensed from the assumptions of a dialectical universe that were mentioned earlier. If a theory is to allow a practice that is particularly conducive to the development of health, it must:

One. Recognize, acknowledge, respect, and account for a totality, or system larger than its parts. If a theoretical approach is likely to be productive for nursing practice it should include, minimally, the concepts of synergy and systems and, optimally, the concept of holism. The nursing literature seems to reflect a fairly consistent understanding of the concepts of synergy and systems and a general agreement about their applicability and utility. Holism, on the other hand, which according to Rogers is "the most difficult construct to comprehend in nursing's conceptual model,"[23] has been popularized to such an extent that it has come to have many different, often inconsistent, and sometimes conflicting meanings. As a means of explanation in the natural and social sciences, holism theorizes at a level that is "irreducibly macroscopic" and in direct contradiction with any idea of individualism.[24] In a comprehensive review of the concept, Mathwig presents holism as generally accepted ontology with powers of regulation and coordination, the ability to establish unity and to assimilate new input with preexisting activities by incorporating such aspects of the whole as relationships, patterns, form, and function.[25]

Nonetheless, the concept of holism continues to suffer from confusing interpretations and the difficulties inherent in its operationalization. Yet it remains an attractive idea for nursing scholarship, as it comes closest to providing a theoretical basis that matches nurses' practical experiences. People do "seem" to be more than their parts. Theories that do not take such totalities into account will find themselves expending considerable energy, that might have been used for greater benefit, in either accounting for the discrepancies between their explanations and realities, distorting an unwieldy and recalcitrant reality into particulate images, or some combination of the two.

Two. Recognize, acknowledge, respect, and account for the incessant change and ongoing development that characterizes all aspects of human phenomena. A theoretical approach that includes equilibrium as a concept or as a desirable goal of nursing intervention would not be as potentially productive for nursing practice as one that so thoroughly integrates the notion of change that it is expected, planned for, manipulated, and exploited towards nursing's ends. More than merely tolerating or accounting for change, theories need to allow that change must be reveled in if human needs are to be served. Theories that present themselves as absolute or definitive, or as the "one best conceptual model for nursing," are not as potentially productive as those that allow the particulars of the situations under study to be the significant factors in selecting among particular change-respecting theories.

CONTRADICTIONS OF THE DIALECTIC

In order that the basic assumptions might be implemented or translated into practice, dialecticians found it necessary to establish certain other conditions, which were developed within the parameters of the first criteria. There are contradictions in working within a holistic universe that are similar but less apparent to those in a dialectical approach to the world that must be addressed at the outset if any theory is to be a more rather than less productive partner for nursing practice. The problems that result from having acknowledged and adopted a holistic or systems view of the world have been discussed at length in the literature and can be grouped into three general categories: (1) whether, in light of the difficulties that are inherent in such activities, even to attempt to study holistic phenomena; (2) whether, in light of the inevitable distortions and misrepresentations that will occur, to continue to study holistic phenomena with inadequate and inappropriate methods within theoretical frameworks that focus on particulate aspects of the larger whole; and (3) how to find a way to adapt or accommodate to holism's "macroscopic imperative."[26]

Obviously, nursing cannot give up study. Most immediately, that would leave practitioners without the necessary theoretical bases for their work; ultimately it would call the profession's existence into question, as it would default on our social contract.[27] While the second option has been the road most taken till now, it is no longer an automatic choice as is evidenced by (1) the question even being posed, when once it was assumed that quantitative research was the way for nursing to achieve legitimacy as a science; (2) the recent rising popularity of qualitative research methodologies; and (3) the heightened consciousness on the part of quantitative researchers and their attention to and analysis of the discrepancies between holistic and systems world views and the particular theories being studied. Nursing scholars who elect to work in either of these last two ways—with qualitative research methods or with an enlightened understanding of the limits of quantitative methods—are accommodating, as individuals and in individual situations, to the "macroscopic imperative." The third possibility for resolving the contradictions provides for such accommodation at the conceptual level. Because such conceptual accommodation saves wear, tear, effort, and energies that could instead be used for further study, it becomes a third criteria for a theoretical approach that would promote, rather than unnecessarily restrict, the development of health potentials.

Three. Once holism is assumed, one must find a way to recognize, acknowledge, respect, and account for the inevitable distortions that occur when the indivisible totality is artificially divided, as is necessary. Such a process is described within a dialectical understanding of reality by the act of *individuation*, which is "simply a matter of carving up the whole in a different manner for a particular purpose."[21:19] I have argued elsewhere that this concept offers nursing scholarship a way out of the theoretical paradox that comes with holism.[26] Given the assumptions of the dialectic, individuation necessarily reflects the identifying characteristics of incessant change and the relational nature of all phenomena. The distinctive benefit of individuation or any similar concept is that it refocuses nursing's attention away from particulate phenomena toward the changing relationships that develop between these discrete entities and the larger system. This leads to a conceptualization that is closer to reality and so is more likely to coexist with a health-promoting practice than one that would restrict such development.

Four. It is a contradiction of the dialectic that the problems inherent in individuation are also the means by which the dialectic continues to grow and develop. Individuated reality is susceptible to the "forces of abstraction," whereby parts are inaccurately perceived as the whole.[21:62] The dangers of misinterpreting such abstractions and developing nursing interventions from such false premises are obviously of concern to nursing scholars seeking to provide the frameworks that will efficiently and effectively promote healthy behavior.

On the other hand, if the forces of abstraction and their dialectical nature are recognized, acknowledged, respected, and accounted for, they have growth potential. Nurses who begin from the premise that such abstractions are the inevitable by-product of the necessary, albeit distorting, individuation of reality will work cautiously and with a healthy suspicion. Nurses who approach reality by *always* searching for the next abstraction and *always* looking for what the present abstraction can tell about both the next distortion and the underlying dynamic are similar to those who revel in change, depend on and utilize it, rather than struggle to control its dynamism. By giving up the false gods of absolute truth and equilibrium, nurses free considerable energies for other purposes, such as promoting, maintaining, and restoring health. Therefore, a theory that provides the means to do so is more likely to coexist with a health-promoting practice than one that unneccessarily restricts such development.

OPERATIONALIZATION OF THE DIALECTIC

These assumptions and contradictions of the dialectic are operationalized through the means by which reality is individuated and through the particular abstractions that are common to all acts of individuation. The means and abstractions are themselves dialectical in nature and so can be expected to reflect the same assumptions and contradictions from which and through which they develop. Therefore, they are additional useful indicators of a theory–practice relationship that is more likely than not to nurture and promote healthy behavior.

Five. Given the assumptions of the dialectic, abstractions occur in an incessant series of individuations that, given the forces of abstractions, are progressively distorting. At the same time, given the infinite number of internal relations developing during any particular phase of the dialectic, a "false consciousness" is created as abstractions move further and further from reality.[28] The process of understanding and explaining phenomena begins by acknowledging (1) that such a false consciousness exists and (2) that it is also dialectical in nature and so exists in relation to the larger whole. Therefore, despite its distortions or falseness, such a consciousness has the potential to reveal aspects of the phenomena that would otherwise remain hidden.

Whether such a potential is realized is a function of whether the researcher analyzes the false consciousness both for how it distorts and for what the act of distorting can tell about the underlying phenomena. This itself is a manifestation of the contradictory nature of the dialectic in that the same phenomena (the false consciousness) can serve both to hide and to reveal. In turn, whether a particular theoretical approach helps or hinders a health-enhancing practice is a function of whether it provides for the conceptualization of a false consciousness.

Six. The specific dialectical relationship between a society's "base" and its "superstructure" is the mechanism by which a false consciousness develops and extends itself, and it is here that the researcher begins in order to uncover and observe as many as possible of the other dialectical relationships that at any moment constitute reality. A society's "base" is the phenomenon considered as its most central individuation: the one to which all others relate most directly; the "superstructures" are those ideologies and social systems that develop from the base and serve to justify and defend its existence.[29:132] The "base" and "superstructure" are themselves individuations that have been isolated from the dialectical process and so manifest the characteristics of incessant development that identify any phenomena as dialectical. They are different in different sociohistorical times.

Perhaps the most noted discussion of this relationship is in the works of Karl Marx, who identified economic relations as the base of a capitalist society and organized social relations, such as legal, political, religious, aesthetic, and philosophical, as the superstructures that support the continued existence and further development of the base.[29:183] A more contemporary analysis is presented by Habermas, who argues that what were once superstructures—science and technology—have become, through the dialectical process, the basic defining individuations of our era, and that the values of empirical science, rationality, and technocratic control have developed into the superstructures of this postindustrial society.[30] Despite these and other differences in the social science literature about what is the "real" base of society and what is a misperception that results from a false consciousness, the existence and dialectical nature of the relationship between base and superstructure is generally accepted.

As with other individuations, the dialectical interaction between base and superstructure has both conservative and liberating potential. If it is not acknowledged, each side of the base–superstructure relationship will be seen as a distinct, nonrelated abstraction, and the superstructure's function of legitimating the base will be obscured. If acknowledged, however, the legitimation process can tell something about both the ideologies themselves and the primary dynamic of the sociohistorical period. In the first instance, the understanding and explanation of these particular phenomena and their relationship to each other and to other less directly related phenomena is unnecessarily restricted and distorted, whereas it is enhanced in the second. Since such understanding and explanation are basic to health-promoting behaviors, there are corollary expectations that nursing theories should provide or allow for the base–superstructure relationship.

Seven. Because the superstructures also show the characteristics of the underlying dialectical process, they exist as a developmental series of incessant, mutually transforming interactions. The amalgam of superstructure phenomena is identified by Gramsci as a society's hegemony, and some of its most critical functions are as a medium for (1) people realizing their potential (becoming freer and healthier), and (2) the development of the relationship between theory and practice and between intellectuals and the general population.[31:323–43,364–5] These two phenomena also share a dialectical relationship of mutually interdependent development.

Grounded in the philosophy of the dialectic, Gramsci argues that human nature is defined by and realized through the interactions between the individual and the natural and social environment. In order to actualize their humanity, individuals must (1) know the range of possible ways they can purposively interact with their environment, and (2) desire and know how to use them. To the extent that they do, they fulfill their potential to be free and healthy. Freedom, therefore, is contingent on the intellectual activity that will develop a world view consistent enough with reality that individuals can effectively participate in their world.

The logical place for intellectual activity is within the theory–practice relationship. Theory and practice, for Gramsci, are both "conceptions of the world," but they differ in that theory affirms in words what practice displays in effective action. Together, the theoretical affirmation and the effective practice develop dialectically through the infinite number of possible relationships existing at any one time in what Gramsci calls an "ensemble of relations." The particular ensemble that is significant to the theory–practice relationship includes the dialectical stages of preconception, awareness, critical reflection, diffusion, and serving as the bases for action. Therefore, the formation of a critical conception of the world is necessary to the development of freedom and, by extension of the previous argument, to health. Thus nursing theories that hope to promote a practice that will also allow such freedom and health need to acknowledge, respect, and use the interdependence of theory and practice.

Eight. Gramsci goes further than simply stating where this liberating activity takes place; he tells us who will do it and how. "Intellectuals," according to Gramsci, are those whose unique social functions predominately revolve around giving coherence to the infinite number of dialectical interactions that are developing at any particular phase in history. By structuring an "ensemble of relations" from which intellectuals and nonintellectuals can choose a course of action that will increase the level of their active participation in their world, intellectuals enhance the development of freedom and health.

But Gramsci is clear that intellectuals who speak only to other intellectuals develop an understanding of the world devoid of the novelty and creativity that is necessary for continued growth, which is found only in the dialectical relationship between the intellectuals and the general population. Since it is the general population that brings unique perspectives that are more attuned to the feeling and passionate aspects of any phenomena, they are a necessary factor in developing as fully comprehensive an understanding of reality as possible.[31:415] Several things can happen at this point. The general population may perceive the intellectuals as a class apart and their pronouncements, therefore, as alien to and with little practical application for the "real world." The intellectuals may differentiate themselves and their work to the extent that the general population is unable or unwilling to invest their passion. Or, a crisis of confidence may occur as world views offer little coherence and people in turn feel overwhelmed by the possibilities before them and powerless to affect their environments.

If unaccounted for, the forces of abstractions will bring us to a point where coherence and passion are seen as separate, disparate entities rather than two interdependent aspects of the same phenomena. Since there is a direct relationship between a recognition that people are an amalgam of knowledge, passion, and understanding and the extent to which people are free and healthy, the nurturance of the dialectical relationship between intellectuals and the general population becomes a necessary condition for freedom and health. Nursing theories would do better to account for this relationship at the outset and thereby have sufficient resources available for health-promotion activities, rather than expending energies as we currently do on the never-ending series of conferences and papers on the gap between nursing education and nursing service.

SUMMARY AND CONCLUSIONS

If it seems that we have come full circle, it is because we have. But with a twist. We have returned to the point where we began with a new, fuller understanding of how to choose between a doer and a thinker. Or, rather, with an understanding of the dialectic that keeps us from being immobilized by what turns out to be a false dichotomy between theory and practice.

If we accept the basic premise that the world is a system of incessant change and progressive development, then certain inferences can be made about the subsystems of such a universe. The relationship between theory and practice, and the separate entities of theory and practice, are three such subsystems. This chapter has presented a framework within which to analyze whether particular theories have been logically inferred from the premise in order to be able to assess their potential for supporting a practice that is consistent with the values and assumptions of the nursing profession.

A theory will be conducive to a practice that will optimize people's health potential to the extent that it accounts for and provides the ways and means to exploit purposively the following eight points:

1. A world view that is somewhere along the continuum of systems to holism.

2. The processes of incessant change and ongoing development.
3. The unavoidable and necessary distortions that accompany any study.
4. The underlying dynamic of the divisions and distortions.
5. The inherent difference between reality and appearances.
6. The mechanisms by which a society's most central concerns are protected.
7. The impact of such protection on society.
8. The critical vitality of the relationship between intellectuals and the general population.

Admittedly, to assess theories in this way might seem an intellectual exercise that is needlessly complex. Furthermore, regardless of the complexity, the exercise itself might seem unnecessary in light of the dialectical inference that a theory that does not prove useful to practice will atrophy. While there is some validity to both these concerns, it depends on two points that nursing cannot dismiss without serious discussion: First, although it is tempting to avoid the dialectic's labryinths, to do so is to avoid the essential nature of a world view that seems most consistent with nursing's world. Second, although theories that are inconsistent with the values and goals of nursing practice will eventually correct themselves, the question is whether people's health can wait until that happens. The profession's responsibility and accountability to the public calls for us to tend and nurture the relationship between nursing theory and nursing practice.

NOTES

1. A. Kaplan, *The Conduct of Inquiry* (New York: Chandler, 1964).
2. M. E. Conway, "Toward Greater Specificity in Defining Nursing's Metaparadigm," *Advances in Nursing Science*, 7 (July 1985): 4.
3. J. Fawcett, "The Metaparadigm of Nursing: Present Status and Future Refinement," *Image*, 16 (1984): 3.
4. J. Flaskerud and E. Halloran, "Areas of Agreement in Nursing Theory Development," *Advances in Nursing Science*, 2 (October 1980): 3.
5. P. L. Chinn and M. K. Jacobs, *Theory and Nursing: A Systematic Approach* (St. Louis: C. V. Mosby, 1983).
6. P. Moccia, "A Study of the Theory–Practice Dialectic: Toward a Critique of the Science of Man," unpublished doctoral dissertation, New York University, New York, 1980.
7. P. L. Munhall, "Nursing Philosophy and Nursing Research: In Apposition or Opposition?" *Nursing Research*, 31 (1982): 178–81.

8. J. M. Swanson and W. C. Chenitz, "Why Qualitative Research in Nursing?" *Nursing Outlook*, 30 (1982): 241–5.
9. M. B. Tinkle and J. L. Beaton, "Toward a New View of Science: Implications for Nursing Research," *Advances in Nursing Science*, 5 (January 1983): 27–36.
10. P. Moccia, "A Further Investigation of Dialectical Thinking as a Means of Understanding Systems-in-Development: Relevance to Rogers's Principles," *Advances in Nursing Science*, 7 (July 1985): 33–38.
11. M. M. Leininger, *Qualitative Research Methods in Nursing* (Orlando, Florida: Grune & Stratton, 1985).
12. H. R. Feldman, "Nursing Research in the 1980s: Issues and Implications," *Advances in Nursing Science*, 3 (October 1980): 85–92.
13. M. C. Smith, "Research Methodology: Epistomologic Considerations," *Image*, 16 (Spring 1984): 42–46.
14. A. I. Meleis, *Theoretical Nursing: Development and Progress* (Philadelphia: J. B. Lippincott, 1985).
15. Committee on Medical Education, New York Academy of Medicine, "Statement on Nursing Education: Status or Service Oriented?" *Bulletin of the New York Academy of Medicine*, 53 (1977): 504.
16. R. Ellis, "Characteristics of Significant Theories." *Nursing Research*, 17 (1968): 217–22.
17. M. E. Hardy, "Evaluating Nursing Theory," in *Theory Development: What, Why, How?* (New York: National League for Nursing, 1978).
18. M. Duffey and A. F. Mullenkamp, "A Framework for Theory Analysis," *Nursing Outlook*, 22 (1974): 570–74.
19. B. J. Stevens, *Nursing Theory: Analysis, Application, Evaluation* (Boston: Little, Brown, 1979).
20. J. Fawcett, *Analysis and Evaluation of Conceptual Models in Nursing* (Philadelphia: F. A. Davis, 1984).
21. B. Ollman, *Alienation: Marx's Conception of Man in Capitalist Society* (Cambridge, England: Cambridge University Press, 1976).
22. B. Ollman and E. Vernoff, *The Left Academy: Marxist Scholarship on Campus*, Vol. II (New York: Praeger, 1985).
23. M. E. Rogers, *An Introduction to the Theoretical Basis of Nursing* (Philadelphia: F. A. Davis, 1979).
24. W. H. Dray, "Holism and Individualism in History and Social Science," *Encyclopedia of Philosophy*, Vol. 4 (New York: Macmillan, 1967), pp. 53–58.
25. G. M. Mathwig, *Holism in the Health Care System*, paper presented at the Nevada League for Nursing, 1978.
26. P. Moccia, "Dialectics of Theory Development," in *Patterns in Education: The Unfolding of Nursing* (New York: National League for Nursing, 1985).
27. American Nurses' Association, *Nursing: A Social Policy Statement* (Kansas City: American Nurses' Association, 1980).
28. G. Lukacs, *History and Class Consciousness: Studies in Marxist Dialectics*, R. Livingstone, trans. (Cambridge, Massachusetts: MIT Press, 1971).
29. K. Marx, "Preface to *A Contribution to the Critique of Political Economy*," in *Karl Marx and Frederick Engels, Selected Works* (New York: International Publishers, 1974).
30. J. Habermas, *Theory and Practice*, J. Viertel, trans. (Boston: Beacon Press, 1973).
31. A. Gramsci, *Selections from the Prison Notebooks of Antonio Gramsci*, Q. Hoare and G. N. Smith, eds. and trans. (New York: International Publishers, 1971).

3

RECONCEPTUALIZING THE ENVIRONMENT

Teresa J. Chopoorian, EdD, RN
Associate Professor
College of Nursing
Northeastern University
Boston, Massachusetts

THE CURRENT STATUS OF THE CONCEPT OF ENVIRONMENT

With few exceptions, nurse theorists have not elaborated upon the concept of environment, even though it is a central element in the nursing paradigm (person, health, nursing, and environment).[1, 2] Nurse theorists regard environment as the immediate surroundings or circumstances of the individual or, as Roy explains, "the constantly changing but often predictable composition of people, places and objects that surround the person."[3:3] Other nurse theorists regard environment as the source of stimuli to which individuals respond or as the interactional field in which individuals accommodate, assimilate, or adjust to the prevailing social mores, customs, and expectations of a society's dominant ideology.[4-7]

Nightingale recognized the environment as the origin of conditions that required critique and action in order to prevent illness and promote health for human beings. Through her famous Blue Book reports, she documented the squalid state of affairs in British hospitals and tried to convince the public and government officials of the need for clean environments.[8] She understood the role played by social, political and economic structures on the health status of British soldiers during the Crimean War. She experienced the consequences herself of acting contrary to the socially prescribed roles of women of her class during the Victorian era. And she recommended that nurses undertake certain measures to protect the environment of the ill person. In recommending that nurses consider "the five essential points in securing the health of houses: pure air, pure water, efficient drainage, cleanliness and light," she brought attention to critical factors external to the patient that influenced the health outcome.[9:24]

When environment is described in the nursing literature, it is primarily regarded as society or the setting to which people adapt or conform. With a tendency to concentrate almost exclusively upon the adaptive capacities of individuals, nursing theories do not encompass explanations for persons or groups who refuse to reject accommodation to environment that present intolerable or unacceptable social, political, or economic circumstances. There are environments that precipitate social or political movements. There are people who refuse to accept perceived injustices or who refuse to adjust or adapt to the society's dominant ideology. Nursing theories do not have an explanation of environment that accounts for prison revolts, riots motivated by racism, or for violence against women, children, and the elderly in society.

Today, in contrast to the past, nurses are not generally observed among those calling for restructuring of societies or for social transformations, even though nurses are eye witnesses to the most deleterious effects of environment on the fate of particular individuals. Nurses observe first-hand the effects of illness in individuals who lack housing, jobs, health care, schooling, and food, basic resources expected by members of a society. Yet it is unusual for nurses to act as advocates for those individuals or groups who refuse to accept the injustices of mainstream ideology. Nursing ideas do not generally encompass a perception of environment as intolerable circumstances for large populations, sometimes for whole societies, intolerable to a degree that precipitates widespread social unrest, labor strikes, popular uprisings, revolutionary movements, or anarchistic states. Yet nursing practitioners continually confront the human responses to the underlying social dynamics of poverty, unemployment, undernutrition, isolation, and alienation precipitated through the structures of society.

Although nurses do examine the root causes of the person's presenting or potential health problem, they usually approach origins of illness or other issues from epidemiological perspectives. That is, the client or patient and other individuals in the community are examined for the causative agents underlying the actual or potential problem. Environmental characteristics, such as demographics and morbidity and mortality rates, are analyzed from the individual or family's specific situation. Factors such as toxic agents, microbes, viruses, or other hazards to health in the individual's environment are considered as effects upon the individual and as threats to the individual's integrity.

Environment is not analyzed as social landscape, as geography. Nursing ideas lack an archeology of the social, political, and economic worlds that influence both client states and nursing roles. In an attempt to establish its unique role, nursing practice has been carried out in the immediate surroundings of the patient. The arena for nursing practice has not reached beyond the immediate milieu of the patient into the dominant social, political, and economic structures that produce behaviors associated with class relationships, power relations, political interests, economic policies, and ideologies such as sexism, racism, ageism, and classism that influence persons in their worlds—behaviors that interfere with health and that eventually cause illness.

In its current state, environment is a rigid, static concept; it does not inform the nursing paradigm in a substantive manner, nor does it foster comprehensive images and relationships. A language to describe the images that constitute environment as a field or as topic of study is missing from the literature of nurse theorists. Environment has not been conceptualized into descriptive units or categories for analysis. Rather, environment, taken for granted as the context of the client and as the setting for nursing practice, remains ambiguous, diffuse, and blurred as a concept, despite the continual reference to it in the language of nursing.

While environment is given attention, it is the concept of the person that holds the paramount place in the conceptualization of nursing by practitioners, researchers, and educators alike. With the focus on person, either as individuals or groups, such as families or communities, nursing is described in relation to the individual's responses to health- or illness-provoking situations. As stated in the American Nurses' Association *Social Policy Statement*, "Nursing is the diagnosis and treatment of human responses to actual or potential health problems."[10:9]

Even the nursing process is constructed upon assumptions about the client as a person, family, or community in that interventions are planned for individuals. Nursing practitioners initiate interventions when individuals have actual or potential health problems that need attention. Nurses respond to situations that need to be ameliorated. Nurses are regarded as problem solvers, the problem being observable and demonstrable in the person or family. Nurses are viewed as health practitioners who assist persons to adjust or adapt to illness. As practitioners, nurses help individuals maintain normal health states, adjust to deviations from normal, and respond to human crises, without necessarily attending to or acting upon the social, political, or economic conditions in the larger society that produce the individual's situation. Nursing practitioners do not generally consider strategies for changing, adjusting, or altering environments; it is persons who adjust, assimilate, or accommodate and nurses who support them in this process.

Persons, not societal structures or institutions, are seen as the focus for change or adaptation. With the individual as the focus for nursing interventions, the environment, as a complex set of structures and relationships, fades into the periphery of nursing's attention and is not treated as an arena for action. In this paper, I suggest that our concept of environment, which centers the individual and places other social phenomena on the periphery, partially explains why nursing practitioners have not assumed such substantive activist roles as consumer, human rights, or women's right advocate; joined other social movements for improving work conditions, for issues of comparable worth, for societal conditions such as unemployment, poverty and racism, or undernutrition; countered the escalation of human rights violations throughout the world; critiqued the distribution of national, state, and local resources when funds are reduced for human services; or participated with grass-roots or professional efforts to point out the potential consequences of foreign or military policies that are founded upon threats of domination through the use of nuclear weapons.

To assume these activist roles, nurses must perceive the

origins of problems that are less attended to when the focus of nursing is the person, who, as the object of intervention, is thought to need adjustment or adaptation. It is surprising that nurses do not express public outrage about the origins of their clients' most serious problems, especially since they are witnesses to the most painful aspects of acute health problems, long-term illness, and the arduous path of rehabilitation. As an example, nurses care for persons in the home and hospital who have cancer and heart and respiratory diseases that are more and more frequently associated with stressful life-styles, hazards in the workplace, and environmental conditions. Exposure to toxic elements, increasing air and water pollution, careless disposal of hazardous materials, lack of attention to workplace hazards, chemical accidents, and the availability of tobacco are examples of conditions that influence health and illness states.[5] While health professionals and the public are increasingly aware of these harmful conditions, approaches to their resolution mean fundamental changes in the high-technology, corporatized structures of industrialized developed countries.

For example, environmental pollution is produced by toxic materials that seep into air and water during the processes of production, storage, and transportation. Toxic materials are the byproducts of chemical and other similar industries. Chemical spills can occur whenever chemicals are produced; illness from careless or even careful exposure to chemicals by workers are always possible. Taking up these issues means entering the sphere of the nation's economic interests, which weigh the costs and benefits of risks to workers and others against considerations of profit and product development. This suggests the need to alter the economic basis of American institutions and organizations, a prospect that would be highly resisted by powerful interests and their political allies.

Lack of a consciousness of environment may also contribute to the peripheral role of nursing practitioners in the larger arena of social, economic, and political affairs in the United States. Nursing practitioners do not regularly lobby or otherwise participate in local or statewide political offices, such as health boards, environmental and sanitation committees, and water and air regulatory bodies. They do not speak out against racism or point out the consequences of environmental pollution. While nursing leaders and nursing organizations have sought to improve conditions for nursing education, practice, and research, most of their efforts to date have been used to further enhance the profession of nursing. Nursing practitioners have not formed strong alliances with consumer groups, such as the elderly, to redress or rectify their problems through social and political action. Nursing practitioners have not looked to the social world, the environment of human experience, for the origin and perpetuation of problems that affect both themselves and their clients. Instead, nurses and the nursing profession tend to look at both the profession and the client as the object of reform or revision.

CONSEQUENCES OF A BLURRED CONCEPT OF ENVIRONMENT

This paramount focus upon the individual or group of individuals is hard to fault, particularly in contrast to other health professionals, who tend to concentrate on parts or pieces of the person. Yet there are consequences for the nursing profession as a result of this concentrated attention on persons and tendency to explain the human condition from the immediate surrounding social world of the individual. Nursing's arena for intervention and action has been restricted or limited to institutionally confined settings. Most nurses practice within organized health services. Access to the persons for whom nurses are ultimately and vitally concerned depends upon institutional relationships. Yet many of the persons who would most benefit from nursing services do not have access to institutions through nurses. And despite the health promotion–disease prevention orientation of nurses, community-based nursing practice centers have not received fiscal support in sufficient amounts to establish new forms of health services.

While individualized attention for persons is not in itself a problem in the diagnosis and treatment of human responses to actual or potential health problems, it does contribute to the tendency of society and the health system to underutilize or misutilize professional nursing personnel. As nurses remain institutionally based in organizations controlled by corporate and profit-motivated interests, they are restricted from broader applications of their knowledge or from the more progressive roles of influence in the larger arena of the social world. Despite the immense value that nurses place on the health and welfare of human beings, professional nursing practitioners have virtually no influence on the development of foreign policy, labor policy, economic affairs, international peace efforts, and the like. Yet societal structures and the human, social relationships that result from the internal dynamics of these structures are processes that influence health or illness states. Even though professional nurses, more than any other health workers, have first-hand and comprehensive knowledge about the health and illness states of persons through immediate experience, they still struggle for a substantive place in the formulation of social, political, and economic policies related to health, education, and social welfare.

The paradigm for nursing intervention, then, the sphere for enactment of the nursing role, is individualized, to a degree privatized, and situationally or institutionally oriented. Nursing roles have been carved out in relation to the person's psychosocial responses to problems, not to the root causes of their problems. As a result, nursing practitioners have focused more on the psychosocial and developmental aspects of health and illness rather than on the sociopolitical and economic aspects of the social world that produce conditions and relationships related to stress, crises, poverty, malnutrition, and illness. In effect nursing's paradigms have led to the production of roles largely confined to institutional settings where clients are housed for treatments mostly provided by nurses but prescribed or initiated by others.

As a result, the social, political, or economic world in which the person is an actor—the environment, the setting of human experience in everyday life—has not been the focus of attention or conceptualized as a field, as a panorama for intervention and action by nurses; at least, not by the typical practitioner of nursing.

POSSIBILITIES OF A RECONCEPTUALIZED ENVIRONMENT

I have made the claim here that concentration upon the person as the central focus of nursing interventions limits nursing practice roles. In addition, societal dynamics continue to reproduce problems and issues that are illness-producing, and in escalating forms. The incidence of cancer, suicide, alcoholism, and violence against women, children, and the elderly is increasing. The most persistent, complex, and deeply obstinate health problems—alcoholism, drug abuse, heart disease, stroke, suicide, malnutrition, and mental illness—which produce the human responses that nurses diagnose and treat, are related to the structure of the social world, the economic and political policies that govern that structure, and the human, social relationships that are produced by the structure and the policies.[11, 12]

A reconceptualization of environment is in order, one that will lead nurses beyond the primacy of their psychosocial orientation to a sociopolitical-economic perspective. In reconceptualizing the environment, a language of descriptive categories, subconcepts, and labels is necessary to share observations, interpretations, and meanings of human and societal processes that constitute the setting and context that influence health and illness states.

Concepts help us to see, to interpret, to make meanings. They are the kernels of thought that lead to theorizing. As Newman suggests, "a concept is an abstraction formed by generalizations from particulars," a way of looking at things.[6:15] As Mitchell says, "concepts are vehicles of thought. They involve mental processes that enable the conceptualizer to identify objects, behavior, feelings, events, phenomena, to recognize commonalities and relationships, to predict outcomes and options and to decide on actions that are appropriate. Concepts are an organization of sub-concepts."[13]

Reconceptualizing environment will further the conceptualizations of health and nursing. A reconceptualization of environment will contribute to the efforts toward a theory of health. Understanding the origins of health or illness and the mechanisms that perpetuate them is a fundamental requirement for a science of nursing. As Hoff suggests, "consideration of origins may or may not include causes." Considering origin suggests that instead of asking "what," we can begin to ask how, under such and such conditions, such and such phenomena occur; in other words, how social, political, economic, and cultural factors and fundamental societal processes and human relations produce health or illness.[14:38]

Throughout this paper, the terms social, economic, and political structures and human, social relations have been used to point out a potential redirection of nursing thought, beyond the immediacy of individual concerns toward larger social, political, and economic concerns. This redirection would not abandon concern for individuals, families, or communities but rather would steer away from the privatizing of problems; that is, the formulation of explanations from the nature and circumstances of specific individuals. This redirection would consider that individuals are a small-scale display of large-scale issues and problems.

In an effort to reconceptualize environment, I suggest here that nurses develop a consciousness of environment as social, economic, and political structures; of environment as human, social relations; of environment as everyday life. These consciousnesses might be considered as potential descriptive categories, as possible labels for subconcepts in a beginning effort to approach environment as the landscape and geography of human, social experience.

These types of categories related to a consciousness of other spheres of the social world are suggested as an example of what is possible when the environment is explored beyond individualized and privatized foci. By considering the dynamics of each and their interrelationships, we may arrive at a more comprehensive view of the internal processes of the social world of human interaction and the infrastructures of organizational and institutional arrangements. The categories suggest what may be possible as frame and focus in a reconceptualized environment. From a consideration of these structural processes, the origins of conditions that support health or militate against it may be better understood.

Following is a brief description of some potential subconcepts, arrived at from a consciousness of social and economic structures, that can inform the concept environment.

ENVIRONMENT AS SOCIAL, POLITICAL, AND ECONOMIC STRUCTURES

The structure of a society's institutions, organizations, and economy produces social life and human, social relations. Attention to a society's social, political, and economic structures refers to a consciousness of the interrelationships between government, private industry, corporate life, philanthropic organizations, social, health, and educational institutions, and everyday life; moreover, attention to these organizations reveals their interconnections and reliance on a common ideology to produce the society's materials, goods, services, and resources.

The United States is characterized by highly bureaucratic forms of organizations and institutions in which centralized power and authority have produced a corporate class and other types of social arrangements that are highly stratified and hierarchical. These arrangements are reproduced in other forms of social interaction and influence the health sector as well. As Waitzkin points out,

> the "corporate class" includes the major owners and controllers of wealth. They comprise 1 percent of the population and own 80 percent of all corporate stocks and state and local government bonds; their estimated median annual income in 1979 was $137,000 to $170,000. The "working class," at the opposite end of the scale, makes up 49 percent of the population. It is composed of manual laborers, service workers, and farm workers, who generally earn $9,100 per year or less. Between these polar classes are the "upper middle class" (professionals . . . comprising 14 percent of the population and earning about $44,600; and middle-level business executives, 6 percent of the population and earning about $28,400) and the "lower middle class" (shopkeepers, self-employed people . . . artisans, comprising 7 percent of the population, earning about $13,700; and clerical and sales workers, 23 percent of the population, earning about $11,700 per year).[11]

Through these structures, some groups have assumed the power and authority to make decisions that influence large sectors of the population. Through these forms of institutional arrangements, efficiency, productivity, and profit have become the measure of worth. Matters related to the production and accumulation of capital by the decision-making sectors are seen as priorities and goals; persons, as workers, increasingly associated with high-technology operations, are regarded as the instruments for achieving the goal.

In quest of these goals, little attention is paid to the quality of human and social experience, and increasingly less attention to the nature of the physical world. Exploitation of workers in the United States and in other countries, hazardous work settings, unfair labor practices, the creation of new classifications of illnesses, and a general fragmentation of social relations are produced from these societal dynamics. As such, the health of various population groups is affected by these societal dynamics; and the health sector, also a system of highly bureaucratized organizations, is a feature of the dominating structures that increasingly are driven by efficiency, profit, and productivity.

For example, research increasingly shows that there are strong causal relationships between smoking and the incidence of heart disease, emphysema, and lung cancer. The U.S. government supports cancer research, funds the National Institutes of Health, publishes warnings to the general public on the dangers of smoking to health, and requires cigarette manufacturers to print health warnings on their products. However, the government also subsidizes the tobacco industry, which produces the product that is believed to be a carcinogen and hence the cause of devastating illness. By attending to environment as social, political, and economic structures, the interrelationships between these structures and the origin of health or illness are better understood.[12,15]

These perspectives are not generally present in the thoughts of practitioners at the bedside, since they are usually preoccupied with the tasks and associated knowledges necessary to carry out chemotherapeutical protocol, or the effects of the potential loss of a family member on the family unit. Thus the origins of illness remain unexplored. Yet the dynamics of social, political, and economic structures continue to produce the conditions leading to illness in persons for whom nurses are responsible.

ENVIRONMENT AS HUMAN, SOCIAL RELATIONS

These social, political, and economic structures also produce human, social relations. Domination, power, and authority or organizational life are reproduced in everyday human interactions. People are surrounded in their everyday lives by a variety of relationships—with family members, with those who are younger, with those who are older, with those who are familiar and with strangers, with those who are perceived as having more or less power, authority, or control.

There are particular characteristics in these relationships that play out the unequal distribution of power seen in organizations between managers and workers and between men and women and then reproduced in everyday interactions between men and women, older and younger persons, children and adults, members of different ethnic and racial groups, friends and coworkers, and administrators and workers. It can be seen that a horizontal or a vertical dimension characterizes these relationships. These dimensions have an internal dynamic of the other being perceived as friendly, near, and equal or as distant, either "up" or "down." For example, we observe that in the United States children are expected to defer to adults, and that adults defer to authority—either the authority of the state, the authority of experts and professionals, or, until recently, the traditional authority and dominance of males, elites, whites.

As Henley suggests, "elements of status, power, dominance, superiority—the vertical dimension of human relations, signalled by our spatial metaphors of 'higher-ups,' 'underlings,' 'being over,' and 'looking up to' is an unattended aspect of human, social relations.[16:2] Henley goes on to say:

> In front of, and defending, the political-economic structure that determines our lives and defines the context of human relationships, there is the micropolitical structure that helps maintain it. This micropolitcal structure is the substance of our everyday experience. The humiliation of being a subordinate is often felt most sharply and painfully when one is ignored or interrupted while speaking, towered over or forced to move by another's bodily presence, or cowed unknowingly into dropping the eyes, the head, the shoulders. Conversely, the power to manipulate others' lives, to take graft, price gouge, or plan the bombing of far-off peasants is conferred in part by others' snapping to attention in one's presence, their smiling, fearing to touch or approach, their following one around for information and favors. These are the trivia that make up the batter for that great stratified waffle that we call our society.[16:3]

Goffman also identified the principle of "symmetric relations between status equals and asymmetric ones between unequals":[16:4]

> Between status equals we may expect to find interaction guided by symmetrical familiarity. Between superordinate and subordinate we may expect to find asymmetrical relations, the superordinate having the right to exercise certain familiarities which the subordinate is not allowed to reciprocate . . . . in American business organizations the boss may thoughtfully ask the elevator man how his children are, but this entrance into another's life may be blocked to the elevator man, who can appreciate the concern but not return it.[16:4-5]

The vertical, hierarchic dimension, and the horizontal dimension that characterizes friendships, intimacies, and closeness between individuals are generally not described as phenomena or considered in their relationship to health or as conditions that produce anxiety, stress, and illness. Racism, sexism, ageism, classism—all products of human, social relations —are not generally regarded as conditions of health or illness.

A consciousness of human, social relations as environment leads to explorations of the relationships between sexism, health, and illness. For example, there is recent evidence that women are increasingly suffering from eating disorders. Psychiatric-mental health nurse specialists are increasingly treating young women with anorexia nervosa and women of all ages who are bulimic. Nurses, in their present person-oriented roles, deal with the human responses to these issues. Yet a more comprehensive concept of environment would question the origins of exploitation of women and other forms of sexism and their relationship to illnesses such as bulimia. A consciousness of human, social relations as the origin of conditions for sexism also leads to deeper understandings of violence directed at women in society.

ENVIRONMENT AS EVERYDAY LIFE

The social world and its structures also make up the framework of everyday life. The everyday life of persons, characterized by their habitual, mundane, routine activities, is not of general interest to practitioners of most disciplines. It is that blur of life, the routinized habits that propel persons from situation to situation until something interrupts the regular. It is what Schutz described as the individual's paramount reality.[17] It is perhaps the least understood or attended to aspect of human experience and perception. However, it is to the experiences of everyday life that persons react and respond. Individuals interpret out of everyday life. They seek direction from the everyday. They act upon meanings from everyday life. It is from everyday life that events or crises, interrupt or reject the routine. As Brittan says:

> Catching buses, going to the toilet, observing traffic rules, going to a pub, eating with knives and forks, talking to one's friends, mowing the lawn, all the mundane activities informing social existence, are not questioned in a systematic manner. Provided nothing interrupts the flow of mundane happenings, there is no apparent need to theorise about the world. For participants, the routinized world is reality, its appearance is not superficial, there is nothing beyond routine because routine is all there is—at least, they do not question its apparent ubiquity. In so far as participants are

not conscious of the ordinariness of everyday routine, they have no need to examine the typicality of the world they live in. But, of course, the world does not stand still, routines are interrupted, personal and social crises infringe on the calm of mundane reality. The ebb and flow of everyday life involves more than routine, it involves consciousness of differences between the boring present and the threatening future, the possibility of pain and suffering, and more appositely, consciousness of the actuality of personal troubles.[18:21]

For example, everyday life for blacks, Asians, and "colored" (mixed race) South Africans is apartheid, a system that constitutionally prohibits them from most of or all of the rights of citizenship. Without the privileges of citizenship, this large majority of the population is denied access to productive employment, appropriate schooling, and adequate health care. Hence, to be a teacher, a nurse, or whatever in South Africa is to witness as everyday life the social, political, and economic privileges of the white minority who control the society's resources while the majority of the population are denied participation. It is from a consciousness of their everyday lives that black South Africans have rejected the dominating structures of their society that have led to the escalated social tensions which are producing structural changes in the society.

As Brittan explains,

the private lives of the white middle class in Johannesburg proceeds as if the world outside was a convenient backdrop to their highly privatised lifestyle, but this is not equivalent to saying they are victims of everyday life, they are deluded by their apparent ability to play middle-class games in which the limits are circumscribed by the definite prescriptions of the law and state.[18:23]

Thus, as Brittan explains, "the routines of everyday life can be grasped in their concrete particularity, and it is in the confrontation between personal troubles and public issues that this concreteness is most apparent."[18:21–22]

A similar perception of a consciousness of everyday life is occurring for many of the people in the countries of Central America. For example, in El Salvador, wealth is concentrated in the hands of a small part of the population of five million. The majority are deprived of basic resources to sustain human life. As a result, more than half of the children suffer from malnutrition; the infant mortality rate is more than 50 percent; in 1975, more than 250,000 families—approximately 39 percent of the population—lived in one-room dwellings; and only approximately 37 percent had access to potable water.[19] It is a consciousness of, a recognition of the relationships between the societal structures and everyday life that have created the social tensions that have moved members of this society to reject the dominance of the existing structures.

Or in Nicaragua, for 50 years before the 1979 revolution, the country operated on what Collins describes as "the logic of the minority, meaning that decisions were made in the interest of, and usually by, the wealthiest 10 percent of the population. As a consequence, the majority of Nicaraguans have been amongst the poorest people in Latin America. The incidence of malnutrition had doubled in the ten years before 1975, crippling the lives of almost 60 percent of children under four years of age."[20:2]

CONCLUSION

This paper suggests that substantive scholarship needs to be directed to the explication of categories like these and others with the goal of describing environment in ways that will uncover new possibilities for nursing practitioners to contribute to the solution of societal problems.

The concept of environment needs to move into a place of prominence in nursing thought. To understand the dilemmas and issues that influence human beings and hence create conditions for health or illness, nurses must reach beyond the privatized concerns of the individual to the surrounding world for explanation and action. Nurses need to turn their attention to the conditions that control, influence, and produce health or illness in human beings. Out of concern for individuals, nurses must look to the larger social world for analysis and explanation. With a perspective of the individual as the particular and the environment as the general, nurses can arrive at more adequate explanations for the origins of individual problems.

NOTES

1. P. L. Chinn and M. K. Jacobs, *Theory and Nursing: A Systematic Approach* (St. Louis: C. V. Mosby, 1983).
2. A. Thibodeau, *Nursing Models: Analysis and Evaluation* (Monterey, California: Wadsworth Health Sciences Division, 1983).
3. B. Randall, M. P. Tedrow, and J. Van Landingham, *Adaptation Nursing: The Roy Conceptual Model Applied* (St. Louis: C. V. Mosby, 1982).
4. J. Fawcett, *Analysis and Evaluation of Conceptual Models of Nursing* (Philadelphia: F. A. Davis, 1984).
5. J. Fitzpatrick and A. Whall, *Conceptual Models of Nursing: Analysis and Application* (Bowie, Maryland: Robert J. Brady, 1983).
6. M. Newman, *Theory Development in Nursing* (Philadelphia: F. A. Davis, 1979).
7. R. R. Parse, *Man-Living-Health: A Theory of Nursing* (New York: John Wiley & Sons, 1981).
8. Cecil Woodham-Smith, *Florence Nightingale* (New York: Atheneum, 1983).
9. Florence Nightingale, *Notes on Nursing: What It Is and What It Is Not* (New York: Dover, 1969).
10. American Nurses' Association, *Nursing: A Social Policy Statement* (Kansas City: American Nurses' Association, 1980).
11. H. Waitzkin, *The Second Sickness: Contradictions of Capitalist Health Care* (New York: The Free Press, 1983).
12. Samuel Epstein, *The Politics of Cancer* (New York: Anchor Books/Doubleday, 1979).
13. P. Mitchell, *Concepts Basic to Nursing Practice*, 2d ed. (New York: McGraw-Hill, 1977).
14. L. A. Hoff, *People in Crisis: Understanding and Helping*, 2d ed. (Menlo Park, California: Addison-Wesley, 1984).
15. H. Waitzkin and B. Waterman, *The Exploitation of Illness in Capitalist Society* (Indianapolis: Bobbs-Merrill, 1974).
16. N. M. Henley, *Body Politics: Power, Sex and Nonverbal Communication* (Englewood Cliffs, New Jersey: Prentice-Hall, 1977).
17. A. Schutz and T. Luckmann, *The Structures of the Life World* (Evanston: Northwestern University Press, 1973).
18. A. Brittan, *The Privatized World* (London: Routledge & Kegan Paul, 1977).
19. T. S. Montgomerey, *Revolution in El Salvador: Origins and Evolution* (Boulder, Colorado: Westview Press, 1982).
20. Joseph Collins, *What Difference Could a Revolution Make? Food and Farming in the New Nicaragua* (San Francisco: Institute for Food and Development Policy, 1982).

Part II

Methodologies

4

QUANTITATIVE METHODS: DESCRIPTIVE AND EXPERIMENTAL

Janet F. Quinn, PhD, RN
Associate Professor
College of Nursing
University of South Carolina
Columbia, South Carolina

In this paper I shall, first, provide an overview of the theory development–research relationship; second, discuss the use of quantitative methods in this enterprise; third, provide an example of the use of the hypothetico-deductive model in the generation of a nursing theory from a nursing conceptual system and describe the use of quantitative, experimental research methods to test a hypothesis derived from this theory; and fourth, identify some unresolved issues related to the theory development–research enterprise.

RESEARCH FOR THEORY DEVELOPMENT

This paper is developed from a perspective wherein theory development is viewed as a two-part enterprise: theory generation and theory testing. Theory development is viewed as incomplete until both of these activities have been accomplished.

The purpose of generating theory in any discipline is to describe, explain, and predict about the phenomenon of concern to the scientist. The primary purpose for testing theory is to determine if there is congruence between the idea of reality which the theory suggests and the empirical evidence of that reality. One wishes to determine if the theory can adequately describe and explain phenomena, with the ultimate goal of being able to predict and control outcomes related to those phenomena. In nursing, we are interested in developing and testing theories that ultimately can assist us in improving nursing care delivery. As we continue to develop our science, we must never forget this goal, however far removed our theories are from actual practice at a given time.

The ideal relationship between nursing theory and research is typically described as a "reciprocal and mutually beneficial one."[1:103] Fawcett refers to the "double helix" of theory and research,[2:49] while Chinn and Jacobs identify the "spiral [that] represents a broadening sphere of knowledge resulting from theorizing that leads to research."[3:151] Thus in this ideal relationship theory directs research, which tests and refines theory, which directs research, and so the spiral goes. This relationship is not only desirable but also critically important to theory development in nursing. Theory must be generated before it can be tested, and research is one very powerful way to do that. Conversely, unless theories are tested through research and found useful in the real world of nursing, they ultimately amount to little more than interesting conceptual fantasies. Quantitative research methods may be and are used in both the generation and testing of theory.

THE THEORY DEVELOPMENT–RESEARCH RELATIONSHIP: A MODEL

Figure 1 presents a model for examining and clarifying the theory development–research relationship. It is presented here to provide a context in which to discuss the use of quantitative research methods in theory development. In this model of the theory development–research relationship there are three interrelated phases: identification of the phenomenon of concern, or the source of research problems; problem conceptualization; and problem solving. In keeping with the scope of this paper, discussion of each of these phases, particularly the first two, is limited to the briefest overview. The reader is referred to texts

FIGURE 1. The Theory–Research Process.

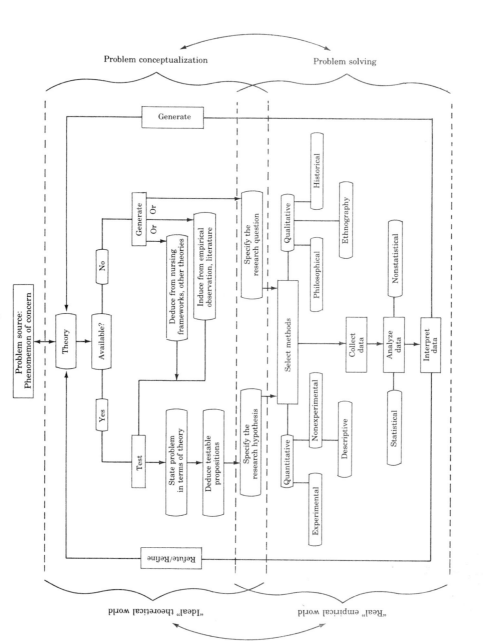

on nursing theory[4-7] for further elaboration of the actual steps involved in theory building and testing, as well as inductive and deductive processes.

PROBLEM SOURCE: THE PHENOMENON OF CONCERN

The phenomenon of concern may be derived out of nursing's metaparadigm[8:84] or from one of nursing's broad conceptual frameworks.[9,10] These are two examples of the elements of nursing's "idea," or theoretical world. If a researcher comes to the business of doing theory development research with the intent of doing so, it is highly probable that this idea world will in fact be the source of the research problem. However, the phenomenon of concern might also arise out of the "real" or empirical world of practice. Nursing research to date is far more often involved with these types of problems than with problems of a more theoretical nature.

PROBLEM CONCEPTUALIZATION

After identifying the phenomenon of concern for research (that is, identifying a broadly stated problem), the researcher begins the problem conceptualization process. First, the researcher determines if there is a theory within which the problem might be examined. The search is for a theory that can describe, explain, or allow prediction related to the phenomenon of concern. The conceptual task involved at this time is to view the problem in the broader context of theory, rather than as an isolated question, interesting as it might seem in its own right. Although it is simply stated, this task can be quite complex and requires discipline, patience, and creativity on the part of the researcher.

Theory Testing. If there is such a theory, then the researcher will engage in testing the theory. Testing of nursing theory is ultimately directed toward determining whether the theory has real-world usefulness, that is, whether it adequately describes the phenomenon of concern to nursing, or adequately explains the phenomena of concern to nursing, including the relationships among and between these phenomena, or that it adequately predicts outcomes of nursing actions related to these phenomena. To test theory, the researcher first states the problem in terms that are consistent with the theory being tested. Through the deductive process, the researcher derives a set of propositions, culminating in the phrasing of a research hypothesis that may be tested in the empirical world. Operational definitions specifying the empirical indicants of the concepts of interest will be determined as part of this process. If this process sounds familiar, it is because it is the traditional, hypothetico-deductive model that is usually assumed to be synonymous with the scientific method in our culture.

Theory Generation. If there is no theory available within which the problem may be examined, the task becomes one of generating theory. This task may be approached in several ways, three of which are represented in Figure 1. The researcher can turn to a broad conceptual framework and use the deductive process to derive a theory, and then proceed as just described in testing the derived theory. Alternatively, the researcher may induce a new theory based on empirical observation, review of the current literature, or educated hunches, which often represent some combination of the two former processes. Again, if theory is generated in this way, then the task of the researcher reverts to theory testing, as can be seen in the model. The third option represented in the model is the generation of theory through the research process. The researcher will review the related literature and pose a research question designed to generate description or explanation of the phenomenon of concern.

Theoretical-Empirical Linkage. At the conclusion of the problem-conceptualization phase of the theory development–research process, the investigator has arrived at either a testable hypothesis or a research question that will guide the problem-solving process. Thus, specification of the research hypothesis or question is both the last step of the problem-conceptualization phase and the first step of the problem-solving phase. It is important to note that the isolated research question or hypothesis does not necessarily convey whether the research is theory generating, theory testing, or neither. Whereas theory-generating research usually contains a research question rather than a hypothesis, theory-testing research often contains questions instead of hypotheses. This is particularly true in the initial attempts to test the theory. Finally, both research questions and hypotheses appear in research with little or no prior problem conceptualization and thus no theoretical affiliation.

It is the research hypothesis or problem that provides the bridge from the theoretical idea world into the real empirical world. If the problem-conceptualization phase has not been adequately addressed, the bridge will be correspondingly weak. The appearance of the bridge does not always accurately reflect its strength, and when one evaluates the bridge, one is wise to examine the underpinnings before assuming structural and functional integrity. Without adequate bridges, problem solving in the real world may occur, but it is exceedingly difficult to return to the theoretical world.

PROBLEM SOLVING

The problem-solving phase consists of the selection and utilization of a set of methods, procedures, and analyses to test the hypothesis or answer the research question. For many, this is the phase to which the term "research" refers. The conceptual task of this phase is to choose the best methods, design, and analyses for the research problem. This task is no less complicated than the task of problem conceptualization. It is, however, a different type of task, with more precise and readily available rules to guide it. It should be obvious that the more clearly the problem has been conceptualized, the easier it will be to proceed through method selection and decisions about design and data analysis.

The culmination of the problem-solving phase is the interpretation of the findings of data analysis. As can be seen from the model, if the research was theory based, then the findings have implications for theory. If a theory was being tested, the findings will indicate refutation or nonrefutation; that is, the hypothesis is rejected or not rejected. A theory is never proved, but a successful or useful theory will survive repeated attempts at refutation. Confidence in the "truth" of a theory is directly related to the number and rigor of tests the theory has survived. The rejection of the null hypothesis of no difference (or conversely the support of the alternative hypothesis) in one study provides direction for further refinement and testing of the theory, and does not result in the conclusion of testing. Thus the notion of replication of research becomes critically important in the development of theory. If the focus of the research was generation of theory, then the findings will be used to inductively identify potentially useful concepts, to describe these concepts, and possibly to develop theoretical statements of relationship between these concepts.

At this point, with the foregoing to provide a context, let us now consider the method-selection aspect of the problem-solving phase in more detail. Since a fuller discussion of qualitative methods appears elsewhere in this book, the following discussion is concerned primarily with quantitative research methods.

METHOD SELECTION

The first decision the researcher must make during the problem-solving phase is the choice of research methods to be used in gathering data about the research problem. In the model presented here, this decision is based on the stated research question or hypothesis and involves making the determination of whether quantitative or qualitative methods are best suited for the purpose of the research. Quantitative research methods are those procedures used in the collection of data that allow for the measurement and description of some variables in numerical terms and that allow the data thus collected to be subjected to statistical analysis. In order for quantitative methods to be used, concepts must be operationally defined as variables and instruments must be available to measure the variables so defined. Note that the model makes a distinction between the *method* used in the research (quantitative or nonquantitative), the *design* of the research study (experimental or nonexperimental), and the method of data *analysis* (statistical or nonstatistical).

Whether the researcher is attempting to generate or test theory, either quantitative or qualitative methods may be utilized. In some cases, the researcher may choose to use some combination of the two approaches. Typically, quantitative methods are used for testing theory whereas qualitative methods are used for generating theory. However, quantitative methods are often used in theory-generating research, and qualitative methods of testing theory have developed out of qualitative investigations. The important point here is that it is not whether or not theory is being generated or tested that determines the method to be used. Rather, it is the research question or hypothesis being posed that governs the selection of a research method.

After making the decision to use quantitative methods, the researcher must choose a study design. If the research question seeks simple description of a phenomenon, a nonexperimental descriptive/exploratory design will be used. Examples of this design include the use of surveys, questionnaires, recurrent observations, and interviews. Given the state of the art in nursing theory development, descriptive/exploratory designs that can lead to empirically derived or tested descriptions of phenomena are very appropriate. If a hypothesis has been formulated to test a theory, a descriptive or experimental design might be used. Several differences between experimental and nonexperimental designs will now be examined.

Experimental and Nonexperimental Designs

The basic distinction between a design that is experimental and one that is not, such as a descriptive design, is the degree of the investigator's manipulation of or intervention into the situation being studied. "The experimental design occurs when the subjects (people or social systems) and conditions (events or situations) to be studied are manipulated by the investigator . . . the key to experimental design is that the investigator assigns subjects to conditions rather than observing them in naturally occurring situations."[11:8] Thus the distinction is not based on the question being asked, the presence of a hypothesis, the number of groups being used, the number of variables being studied, the type of data being collected, or the statistics being utilized to analyze that data. Random assignment to conditions that can be manipulated by the investigator is the sine qua non of experimental design. Without either of these two factors, the design is other than experimental.

Through the processes of random assignment and investigator manipulation of the independent variable, experimental designs allow the researcher to determine whether or not there is a causal relationship between the variables being studied. Support (or nonrefutation) of the hypothesis tested by means of a rigorous experimental design engenders considerable confidence in the theory from which the hypothesis was derived. Replication with similar results adds to that confidence.

Because of the rigor of the design, the experiment is generally considered to be the exemplification of the scientific method: the standard for the conduct of scientific inquiry against which all other approaches are compared and judged. Whether this perspective is useful or not to the development of nursing science is a matter of some debate in recent nursing literature.

In contrast to experimental design, in which the researcher has maximum control, is the nonexperimental design, which is characterized by its lack of manipulation and randomization. The descriptive/correlational approach is one type of nonexperimental design. In correlational studies the relationship between two or more variables is explored, as is true in the classic experiment. However, there is no manipulation of the variables. This design is used when manipulation of the independent variable is not possible, not ethical, or not required by the level of the research question or hypothesis. Nurse researchers have used these designs to test the conceptualizations of reality provided by a variety of nursing frameworks and theories. Fawcett lists examples of research that has been derived from conceptual frameworks.[8:86] Most of the studies cited are descriptive. Hypothesized relationships have been tested primarily through the use of questionnaires, records, or structured interviews that measure the incidence or "amount" of some attributes, traits, or characteristics.

Descriptive studies can establish that one or more variables appear to exist in the real world, as defined by the theory, or that two variables appear to be related to each other. A descriptive study cannot be used to draw causal inferences about the relationship (for example, that one of the variables causes or probably causes the variance in the other variable, or that manipulation of one variable will probably lead to change in the other variable). This is, of course, the major weakness of the descriptive design. When the hypothesis of a descriptive study is supported such that there is an apparent relationship between one or more variables, the theory from which the hypothesis was derived may be considered to be not necessarily wrong. The theory is not supported per se, because alternative theories or explanations for the existence of the phenomenon have not been ruled out, as they are in well-designed experimental studies. But the evidence that the phenomenon, the predicted relationship, has indeed been observed to occur in the empirical world means that the theory that postulates such a relationship is not necessarily wrong.

This is a very useful finding, not for making causal inference, of course, but for encouraging the researcher to continue with additional studies to further describe and explain the phenomenon. Armed with the information that the theory is not necessarily wrong, the investigator might choose to design an experimental study such that the theory is subjected to more rigorous testing and a more precise understanding of the nature of the relationship may be determined. If, on the other hand, a theory allows for the conclusion that certain variables should be related and descriptive studies are unable to demonstrate any relationship between them, then either the theory is wrong or the tools being used for measurement are not adequate or appropriate. The negative finding gives the researcher clear direction for future theory refinement and research. Perhaps the most useful contribution that descriptive studies can make to theory testing is thus to provide instances of nonconfirmation.

The most common error that researchers make in discussing implications of descriptive studies is to infer that there is a causal relationship between the variables studied. This inference is not always explicit, but rather is implicit in statements such as "the implications for nursing practice are that the nurse should do X with patients who manifest Y." The leap from description to prescription is a dangerous one, yet we ourselves often force nurse researchers to make this leap by insisting that every study have immediately recognizable "implications for practice." Often the only legitimate implications of a descriptive, theory-generating, or theory-testing study are for more study.

THEORY-TESTING RESEARCH: AN EXAMPLE

Following is an example of a study that was conducted to test a theory that was deductively derived from a nursing conceptual framework using an experimental design. The full report of this study has been published elsewhere.[12,42] An explicit and detailed description of the theoretical development of the study is included here as an example of the deductive model of theory generation and the quantitative, experimental research approach to theory testing. While this example is not without flaws, it is one of very few studies that appear in the published literature as explicit tests of nursing theory.

PROBLEM SOURCE

The study represents the interests of the author in (1) exploring the phenomenon of therapeutic touch as a nursing intervention consistent with nursing's humanistic values and holistic perspective, and (2) testing the conceptual system developed by Martha Rogers.[13]

PROBLEM CONCEPTUALIZATION

A review of literature relevant to therapeutic touch revealed several findings that provided direction for study. First, the focus of all prior studies, both within and outside of nursing, was the documentation of outcomes of the laying on of hands and the therapeutic touch processes. Thus the central question in each of these studies was "Does the treatment have an effect?"

Second, there was an inconsistency in the method used during the treatment process. In early studies of the laying on of hands, the healer physically touched his human subjects. When plants and animals were studied, however, there was no direct physical contact between the healer and the subjects. In therapeutic touch studies, the practitioner always placed her hands directly on the subjects and thus had direct physical contact with them. In clinical practice with therapeutic touch, clinicians often do not physically touch the person they are treating.

Third, previous investigators had all postulated an explanatory theory, namely, that during the healing act there was some kind of transfer of energy between the healer and the subject, and that this energy exchange was responsible for the outcome of the treatment. Both Grad and Smith arrived at this theory inductively, that is, based on their research observations of the healing process and outcomes involved in laying on of hands.[14:484,15:48] Krieger accepted this theory and then supported it with similar theories from her study of the Eastern literature.[16:12] This theory was accepted as an untested assumption in all studies of laying on of hands and therapeutic touch that followed.[17-20]

It is important to note that although an explanatory theory had been generated through the research process, no empirical tests had yet been undertaken that were designed to test that theory. Research continued to focus on the description of outcomes of the intervention rather than on further explication of the underlying mechanisms responsible for those outcomes. Since the phenomenon of healing through laying on of hands or therapeutic touch was essentially unstudied from a scientific perspective, this was probably appropriate. It would make little sense to ask "How does it work?" before there has been any research evidence that indeed there is some effect to be explained.

Theory Generation. The focus of my study became initial explication of the "how" of therapeutic touch. How can we explain the phenomenon? Since a goal of the research was to examine the phenomenon of therapeutic touch within the Rogerian conceptual system, I derived an explanatory theory out of that conceptual system rather than accepting the inductively determined theory from another discipline. The deductive process described by Blalock and amplified by Newman was utilized to accomplish this task.[7,21] Specifically, relevant axioms (untested or untestable assumptions) of the Rogerian conceptual system were first identified. Then a set of theorems was derived, and out of these theorems, a testable hypothesis was derived. The axioms, theorems, and hypothesis follow. They have been written with the deductive language intact to illustrate the logical, conceptual process that one uses to deduce theory and then to derive from that theory a testable hypothesis.

Axioms of the Rogerian Conceptual System. If it is true that:

1. People are open systems, and that
2. People are irreducible, four-dimensional, negentropic energy fields, and that
3. The environment is an irreducible, four-dimensional, negentropic energy field, and that
4. Persons interact with their environments by means of a rhythmic flow of energy waves, and that
5. Person-to-person interaction is person-environment interaction, and that
6. Change in the human field is an outcome of the continuous, mutual process between human and environmental fields, then it must also be true that

Derived Theorems

1. Therapeutic touch, as a person-to-person interaction, is an energy interaction between two human fields, and if this is true, then it must also be true that
2. The effects of therapeutic touch are outcomes of an energy interaction between "healer" and "healee," and if this is true, then it must also be true that
3. Physical contact between "healer" and "healee" is not necessary for therapeutic touch to have an effect, and if this is true, it must also be true that

4. Therapeutic touch done without physical contact will have the same effects as therapeutic touch done with physical contact.

The reader will note that the first two theorems that were derived from the axioms are not directly testable, and that the second derived theorem is, in fact, the theory proposed by earlier investigators. Thus it becomes obvious that an identical theory may be determined through either the inductive or deductive process. This is important, since often the assumption is made that theories are generated through induction and tested through deduction. When one is working with the broadest of conceptual frameworks, as we are in nursing, it is quite likely that most of our theories will be arrived at deductively, or through some inductive-deductive interactive process, if they are to relate to those frameworks.

Theory Testing. The theory that the effects of therapeutic touch are outcomes of an energy interaction between "healer" and "healee" thus became the theory to be tested through further derivation of theorems and, finally, through derivation of a testable hypothesis from theorem 4. To test this theorem, a known outcome of therapeutic touch with physical contact was selected as an indicant of the effectiveness of therapeutic touch without physical contact.

Derived Hypothesis. It was hypothesized that:

There will be a greater decrease in posttest state anxiety scores in subjects treated with noncontact therapeutic touch than in subjects treated with noncontact.

PROBLEM SOLVING

An experimental design was developed to test the hypothesis. The steps of the noncontact therapeutic touch intervention were specified in the form of an operational definition, as were the steps in the control treatment of noncontact. The control treatment was an exact mimic of the experimental treatment, performed by nurses who did not know how to administer therapeutic touch. Sixty hospitalized cardiovascular patients were randomly assigned to either the experimental or control group, and all subjects completed the State Anxiety Inventory[22] before and after the intervention. Data were analyzed by computing a first order semipartial correlation (part correlation) between treatment group (dummy coded) and posttest score, partialing pretest score out of posttest score. The hypothesis was supported at the .0005 level of significance.

Alternative explanations for the findings other than that postulated by the theory being tested were explored. For example, the study groups were compared on demographic variables such as age, sex, race, and religion and were found to be similar. Thus this alternative explanation for the results was not viable. Placebo effects and the effects of person were ruled out as viable alternative explanations of the results through the use of the control group. Such effects should have occurred in both groups if they were operative. Findings were interpreted as supportive of the theory that the effects of therapeutic touch were outcomes of an energy exchange between the "healer" and the "healee." To place this interpretation in the language of theory development, the study provided an instance of nonrefutation of the theory.

CONCLUSIONS

In this paper the ideal relationship between theory development and research was described, and a model that illustrates this ideal relationship was presented. Within the model, an idea world and an empirical world were identified. Having explored the model, and the ideal relationship, it is now appropriate to acknowledge that both are part of the idea world of nursing, rather than the real world. The need for a linkage between nursing theory and nursing research has been discussed extensively in the nursing literature. Yet most nursing research to date is problem-solving research; that is, research that lacks problem conceptualization in the context of theory development. Very few nursing research studies are designed explicitly to generate or test nursing theory.[23] In an entire issue of the journal *Advances in Nursing Science* devoted to testing of nursing theory, one article out of seven was is in fact a description of research that tested a nursing theory.[24]

One can note an increase in the number of published research reports that describe a theoretical framework for study. Yet these frameworks are rarely being tested, and sometimes they are tangential to the problem being investigated. The extent of reference back to the theoretical framework when the study findings are being discussed is a good indicator of how closely the study is linked to theory development. More often than not in contemporary nursing research literature, this reference is absent. The result of this situation is that "with some exceptions, nursing's current theory is rationally or deductively arrived at, with few empirical verifications."[25] Thus, in spite of a proliferation of nursing research, nursing has little tested and supported theory to guide practice, education, and further research.

There are many possible explanations for this. One is that nursing is not in need of a distinct set of theories for its continued practice and research. Is it possible that the only nurses who require nursing theory are nursing theorists? Could it be true that the urgency to develop nursing theory has more to do with the status of nursing as an academic discipline than it does with nursing as a practice profession? Perhaps nursing theory is essential only to justify our continued presence on the university campus, particularly in graduate schools. While these statements are to some degree merely rhetorical, they may not always be so. If the research literature in nursing does not soon begin to reflect our supposed commitment to a theory development–research enterprise, these are only some of the questions we must be prepared to respond to. At some point, nursing must be able to justify the continued support of nursing research by identifying the body of knowledge that has been and is being developed through that process. When research takes place outside of the theory development framework, it is isolated and thus can contribute little to a body of nursing knowledge.

There are a multitude of unresolved issues related to the theory development–research process. Following are discussions of a few of these.

ISSUES RELATED TO THE PROBLEM SOURCE:
PHENOMENA OF CONCERN

What are the appropriate phenomena of concern for nursing theory development? Fawcett has postulated that nursing has evolved a metaparadigm that defines the phenomenon of interest for nursing as "person, environment, health and nursing."[8:86] Should there be a universal acceptance of these concepts as the foundation for nursing theory development? Should the problems for nursing research derive from the idea world of nursing or from the real world of clinical practice?

Issues Related to Problem Conceptualization

What are appropriate activities of nurse theorists and researchers for the future of theory development in nursing? Should they be attempting to: (1) develop nursing theory out of a variety of existing nursing conceptual frameworks and test the derived theories; (2) work toward acceptance of one conceptual framework for nursing from which to derive nursing theory; (3) generate new nursing conceptual frameworks from which to derive and test new nursing theories; (4) inductively generate theory out of empirical observation or descriptive study; (5) generate theory from the frameworks of related disciplines and then test them in the real world of nursing; (6) accept established theories of other disciplines and test them in the real world of nursing? Is choice between these options necessary, or do we require all of them for nursing theory development?

Issues Related to Problem Solving

Are there some research methods that are better suited than others for use in the theory development–research enterprise? Are quantitative methods appropriate for the study of the phenomena of concern to nursing? How might we increase the reliability and validity of the measurement of the complex variables we are concerned with? Should nursing researchers be attempting to develop new research methods specific to the investigation of nursing problems? Is the experimental design, with its explicit assumptions of causality, appropriate for the study of nursing problems? Should all nursing research be theory development research? What is the value of problem-solving research; that is, research that lacks a clearly defined theoretical linkage?

While there remain many unanswered questions related to the theory development–research relationship, the relationship remains critical to the development of nursing's scientific body of knowledge. Quantitative research methods are powerful tools for both the generation and testing of nursing theory.

NOTES

1. D. Polit and B. Hungler, *Nursing Research: Principles and Methods*, 2d ed. (Philadelphia: J. B. Lippincott, 1983).
2. J. Fawcett, "The Relationship between Theory and Research: A Double Helix," *Advances in Nursing Science*, 1 (October 1978): 49–61.

3. P. L. Chinn and M. K. Jacobs, *Theory and Nursing* (St. Louis: C. V. Mosby Company, 1983).
4. L. O. Walker and K. C. Avant, *Strategies For Theory Construction in Nursing* (Norwalk, Connecticut: Appleton-Century-Crofts, 1983).
5. B. J. Stevens, *Nursing Theory: Analysis, Application, Evaluation*, 2d ed. (Boston: Little, Brown, 1984).
6. P. L. Chinn, *Advances in Nursing Theory Development* (Rockville, Maryland: Aspen, 1983).
7. M. Newman, *Theory Development in Nursing* (Philadelphia: F. A. Davis, 1979).
8. J. Fawcett, "The Metaparadigm of Nursing: Present Status and Future Refinements," *Image*, 16 (Summer 1984): 84–87.
9. J. Fitzpatrick and A. Whall, *Conceptual Models of Nursing* (Bowie, Maryland: Robert J. Brady, 1983).
10. J. Fawcett, *Analysis and Evaluation of Conceptual Models of Nursing* (Philadelphia: F. A. Davis, 1984).
11. P. E. Spector, "Research Designs," Sage University Paper Series on Quantitative Analysis in the Social Sciences, 07-023 (Beverly Hills: Sage Publications, 1981).
12. J. F. Quinn, "Therapeutic Touch as Energy Exchange: Testing the Theory," *Advances in Nursing Science*, 6 (January 1984): 42–49.
13. M. Rogers, *An Introduction to the Theoretical Basis of Nursing* (Philadelphia: F. A. Davis, 1970).
14. B. Grad, "A Telekinetic Effect on Plant Growth II," *International Journal of Parapsychology*, 6 (June 1964): 484.
15. J. Smith, "Enzymes Are Activated by the Laying-On of Hands," *Human Dimensions*, 2 (March 1972): 46–48.
16. D. Krieger, "The Response of In-Vivo Human Hemoglobin to an Active Healing Therapy by Direct Laying-On of Hands," *Human Dimensions*, 1 (January 1972): 12–15.
17. D. Krieger, "Healing by the Laying-On of Hands as a Facilitator of Bioenergetic Change: The Response of In-Vivo Human Hemoglobin," *Psychoenergetic Systems*, 1 (January 1974): 121–29.
18. D. Krieger, "Therapeutic Touch: The Imprimatur of Nursing," *American Journal of Nursing*, 4 (May 1975): 660–62.
19. P. Heidt, "Effect of Therapeutic Touch on Anxiety Level of Hospitalized Patients," *Nursing Research*, 30 (January 1981): 32–37.
20. G. Randolph, "The Differences in Physiological Response of Female College Students Exposed to Stressful Stimulus when Simultaneously Treated by Either Therapeutic Touch or Casual Touch," doctoral dissertation, New York University, New York, 1979.
21. H. Blalock, *Theory Construction* (Englewood Cliffs, New Jersey: Prentice-Hall, 1969).
22. C. Spielberger, R. Gorsuch, and R. Lushene, *STAI Manual for the State Trait Anxiety Inventory* (Palo Alto: Consulting Psychologists Press, 1970).
23. J. Fawcett, "Contemporary Nursing Research: Its Relevance for Practice," in N. L. Chaska, ed., *The Nursing Profession: A Time to Speak* (New York: McGraw-Hill, 1983).
24. "Testing of Nursing Theory," *Advances in Nursing Science*, 6 (January 1984), entire issue.
25. S. R. Gortner, "The History and Philosophy of Nursing Science and Research," *Advances in Nursing Science*, 5 (January 1983): 1–8.

5

QUALITATIVE METHODS: PHENOMENOLOGY

Carolyn J. Oiler, EdD, RN
Associate Professor
College of Nursing
Villanova University
Villanova, Pennsylvania

INTRODUCTION

In the dominant paradigm for nursing research at this time, reality is dichotomized as objective or subjective. The source of this dichotomy is in a focus on an external reality, an existence of things and others independent of the subject who experiences them. Subjectivity is viewed as a private and personal reading of reality that is given to error. Based on this foundational view of the nature of reality, nursing has adopted the scientific aim of isolating cause–effect patterns in nursing situations. Ultimately, we aspire toward control in order to produce predetermined outcomes.

Patient or client subjectivity is valued in our scientific endeavors in two ways: as a data source and as an outcome variable in nursing. In our focus on an external reality, we direct our observation to the world around us as object. Both the client's and the nurse's subjectivity are also treated this way in a scientific stance that narrows our vision of what is real.

There is a basic inconsistency between this scientific perspective and nursing's concern with clients and other nurses as fellow existences in a shared world. Conflict is generated for us in several ways. First, recognition of the nurse–patient relationship as the medium of care competes with scientific devaluing of the nurse's subjectivity in the caring process. Second, nurses suffer the tension of a scientifically polarized reality, which drives subjective experience underground and deprives nurses of control over their realities. Third, awareness of their realities is narrowly confined in the requirements of the professional role, and a gap emerges between their realities as lived and the facts about these realities offered in scientific comment. Fourth, a narrow vision of what it is that happens in experience leaves nurses with unexplained dimensions of reality. And lastly, in order to preserve objective detachment in nursing situations and some sense of integrity for themselves, nurses withdraw from and deny their awareness. This deflects us from values that center nursing as a humanizing influence in the health care system.

The prevailing view of subjectivity in nursing establishes a need to explore other ways of thinking about what is real, so that more in nursing might be considered real in a scientific sense. Phenomenology is a philosophy, a method, and a general approach or orientation that might be interpreted in nursing in efforts to resolve these conflicts. Phenomenology is quintessentially a human interest; a consuming attention to people in their involvement in the world. For nursing, this attention is directed to such phenomena as clients' involvements with their families, with health care technologies, with health care agencies, and with events such as diagnosis, surgery, and discharge. Considered broadly, phenomenological philosophy provides a framework for a variety of qualitative research approaches to phenomena such as these. Although this chapter is focused on phenomenological method, the openness of the philosophy can be capitalized upon to stimulate interest in qualitative research generally.

The qualitative tradition in the social sciences is most easily recognized in sociology and anthropology, with their explicit concerns for the cultural and social realities lived through by people. There is an integral focus on the meanings people attach to objects and others in the environment, and these arise from, and subsequently guide, their interactions with them.

Coming to know a culture is to understand, bit by bit, what it is to be a part of that culture. The anthropological method of participant observation incorporates this premise by placing the researcher *within* the phenomenon under study. This sharp departure from the stance assumed in the positivistic research approach reflects a fundamental difference in the philosophical base of qualitative researchers. This difference is in the attention afforded subjectivity as well as the meanings "subjectivity" has for them.

Wherever one finds the participant-observer technique in research, or efforts to identify sources of data and to design data collection methods that adhere closely to the subject's natural presentation of his experience, or candid discussions by the researcher concerning her subjective sense of what transpired during the project, there is evidence of a qualitative influence on research designs. It is not unusual to read research reports that have a qualitative flavor in the breadth of the variable under study or in the design or analysis of data.

In fact, empirical studies are formally acknowledged as being born of researcher subjectivity both in the creative impulse leading to the study and in such methodological concerns as deciding on operational definitions and selecting instruments when there are multiple possibilities. In this sense, there is no absolute distinction between quantitative and qualitative methodologies. Nevertheless, there are clearly two separate traditions with disparate philosophic assumptions. It is important to recognize these differences and to accept their irreconcilable nature. This does not necessarily lead to destructive conflict in nursing or in any other discipline that embraces more than one paradigm. Rather, open acceptance of contrasting paradigms preserves the advantages and unique perspectives of both.

In the belief that the differences in qualitative research approaches enrich nursing, the prevalent philosophical themes that provide a grounding for these research efforts will be described. Phenomenological method will then be focused in a presentation gleaned primarily from the works of phenomenologist Maurice Merleau-Ponty. The historian of the phenomenological movement, Herbert Spiegelberg, serves as a guide through the multiple schools of thought within phenomenology in an identification of commonalities in the method. Major interpretations of the method in the United States are then briefly described, followed by an overview of selected phenomenological studies by nurses. The chapter concludes with a discussion of how phenomenological method can be applied in nursing research through the author's interpretation of principles that inhere in phenomenological philosophy. Nurse researchers are encouraged to explore the method freely, ferreting out techniques that disclose nursing phenomena faithfully, toward the end that these phenomena can be better understood.

THE PHENOMENOLOGICAL PERSPECTIVE: PRIMARY THEMES

The aim of phenomenology is to describe experience as it is lived by people. The concern in phenomenological studies is to give phenomena a fuller and fairer hearing than empiricism accords them. Phenomenology clearly emerged, and is evolving, as a protest against reductionism and the sense-organ bias constructed in the nineteenth century[1:656] In essence, phenomenologists hold that human existence is meaningful and of interest only in the sense that we are always conscious of something. In this view, pure consciousness, the "I am," is not meaningful. Rather, "I am" a nurse, or "I am" aware of having many patients to care for, or "I am" interested in knowing more about this client.

Merleau-Ponty has described phenomenology variously as the study of essences, a transcendental philosophy that questions facts about our world in order to understand the world more adequately, and a philosophical stance or position that attempts to describe experience as it is lived without concern for how it came to be the way it is.[2:59] The causal explanations and interpretations of scientists and historians are distinguished in this way by the qualitative researcher's belief that people and the world can be understood only through an account that discloses their contacts with the world.

There are in the language of phenomenological philosophy key concepts that bring us closer to understanding the qualitative style of studying the world. Consciousness, or one's presence to the world, and modes of awareness, or one's ways of being conscious—our expressions of consciousness—are phenomenological themes that assist us in understanding this approach to knowledge.

CONSCIOUSNESS AND EMBODIMENT

Consciousness, particularly in the health disciplines, is commonly understood to mean sensory awareness of and response to the environment. Philosophically, this meaning is expanded to include existence generally. Consciousness is life; it is existence in the world through the relations of bodily systems. Merleau-Ponty rejects the Cartesian explanation of consciousness as an interiority that establishes a subjective and an objective world:

> There can be no doubt at all that I think. I am not sure that there is over there an ashtray or a pipe, but I am sure that I think I see an ashtray or a pipe. Nor is it in fact as easy as is generally thought to dissociate these two assertations and hold, independently of any judgment concerning the thing seen, the evident certainty of my "thought about seeing"? On the contrary, it is impossible.[3:374]

Merleau-Ponty reasons that this idea of consciousness as inner existence, independent of the world in which it exists, is false on the grounds that the thought of seeing an ashtray or pipe is possible only because in one's history, one has had this experience. He explains:

> The world is not what I think, but what I live through. I am open to the world, I have no doubt that I am in communication with it, but I do not possess it; it is inexhaustible.[3:xvii]

The fact of the world and the fact of consciousness coincide and are never doubted. All acts of consciousness—remembering, judging, dreaming, and so on—are possible because we are present within the world. This is a critical consideration in Merleau-Ponty's phenomenology. It recognizes consciousness as simultaneous contact with the world and with oneself. The idea of a subjective and objective world is eliminated in this conception.

The world is assumed; experience in it and knowledge of it, however, always come through the subjectivity of being-in-the-world. Knowing oneself in self-consciousness and knowing the world are contingent on one's presence in the world. There cannot be two views of reality—the view is always the subjective one of presence in the world. It is an inseparable dimension of reality as it can be known to man. The appearance of phenomena expresses this welded relationship of subject and object, and is the first or fundamental reality upon which our sciences and understandings are built.

How is it that consciousness thus conceived can be explained? If consciousness is being-in-the-world, how does that become possible? The concept of embodiment explains how this relation between subject and object occurs. Man's body is his natural access to the world. Sensation, sexuality, language, and speech are all expressions of our existence, and all are constituted, concretely, in a bodily reach toward the world.

Merleau-Ponty regards one's body as one's point of view upon the world. The body as access to the world produces for the subject what Merleau-Ponty refers to as one's "gaze." This means that consciousness is expressed in a particular manner of approach to the world; and the approach, or gaze, is brought into being by one's bodily existence in the world.

Elaboration on the idea of human gaze will move us forward in understanding Merleau-Ponty's concept of embodiment:

> Even if I know nothing of rods and cones, I should realize that it is necessary to put the surroundings in abeyance the better to see the object and to lose in background what one gains in focal figure, because to look at the object is to plunge into it, and because objects form a system in which one cannot show itself without concealing others. . . . In normal visions . . . I direct my gaze upon a sector of the landscape, which comes to life and is disclosed, while the other objects recede into the periphery and become dormant, while, however, not ceasing to be there. Now, with them, I have at my disposal their horizons, in which there is implied, as a marginal view, the object on which my eyes at present fall. . . . The object-horizon structure, or the perspective, is no obstacle to me when I want to see the object; for just as it is the means whereby objects are distinguished from each other, it is also the means whereby they are disclosed.[3:67–68]

Merleau-Ponty has outlined the determinants of human experience in these few words. Concretely, we are able to experience the world through our bodies. We bodily assume a position in the world, which in turn determines the horizon–object structure, both spatially and temporally, that is available to us. We are able to focus, to be conscious of, one object over against others in a figure–ground relationship of our choosing.

The human gaze reveals just that aspect of the object accessible through one's bodily involvement in the world in space and in time. Human experience and human reality are always perspectival in this sense. It is important to recognize here, however, that the subject's biography, his past experience, his knowledge of the world, qualifies his gaze by positing other aspects of the object.

When I look at the lamp on my table, I attribute to it not only the qualities visible from where I am, but also those which the chimney, the walls, the table can "see"; but back of my lamp is nothing but the face which it "shows" to the chimney. I can therefore see an object insofar as objects form a system or a world, and insofar as each one treats the others round it as spectators of its hidden aspects and as guarantee of the permanence of those aspects.[3:68]

In this way, a perspective on the world is formed. It is not pure experience but an interpreted experience that constitutes reality.

Alfred Schutz, another phenomenologist, contributes to an understanding of expressions of consciousness in human perspectives in the world:

The origin of all reality is subjective, whatever excites and stimulates our interest is real. To call a thing real means that this thing stands in a certain relation to ourselves. . . . Our primitive impulse is to affirm immediately the reality of all that is conceived, as long as it remains uncontradicted. But there are several, probably an infinite number of various orders of realities, each with its own special and separate style of existence. James calls them "sub-universes" and mentions as examples the world of sense or physical things (as the paramount reality), the world of science, the world of ideal relations, the world of "idols of the tribe," the various supernatural worlds of mythology and religion, the various worlds of individual opinion, the worlds of sheer madness and vagary. The popular mind conceives of all these sub-worlds more or less disconnectedly, and when dealing with one of them forgets for the time being its relation to the rest. But every object we think of is at last referred to one of these subworlds.[4:207]

Schutz explains that it is the direction of consciousness in the world that determines what reality is operative at any given point in time. Referring to this as "attention to life," man chooses reality in this sense by defining meaning in the objective world.

Although there are multiple realities in our shared world, the "paramount reality of the world of sense" cited above is the normal life of consciousness that is expressed within or on the world. The reality of experience is taken for granted, and shifting perspectives are assumed as dictated by one's biography and by the practical need to achieve chosen purposes in the world. The world is both the place where consciousness expresses itself and the object of one's consciousness.

Schutz explains that in the natural attitude, the world as experienced and interpreted by our predecessors is handed down to our own experience and interpretation. In the fashion of layers, a current experience is shaped by a stock of previous experiences and interpretations—one's own and that of one's parents and teachers. The natural attitude, a type of mode of consciousness, presents us with interpreted experience.

The natural attitude characterizes most of our existence. Unquestioned as reality, we assume that the meanings brought to the world coincide with an absolute, objective reality. Other realities, arising from other modes of consciousness, and different attentions to life, presenting other meanings, are incompatible.[4:229-32]

Being-in-the-world, or presence, is inseparable from consciousness. Consciousness is always *of* something. Through the body we have access to the world where consciousness expresses itself in various attentions to life. We know of being only through our involvement with certain objects. Merleau-Ponty describes this involvement as embodiment, meaning that the body is caught up in the world; and through it, consciousness finds expression in thought, feeling, speech, sensing, judging, remembering, and so on:

> Visible and mobile, my body is a thing among things; it is caught in the fabric of the world, and its cohesion is that of a thing. But because it moves itself and sees, it holds things in a circle around itself. Things are an annex or prolongation of itself; they are incrusted into its flesh, they are part of its full definition; the world is made of the same stuff as the body. This way of turning things around, these antinomies, are different ways of saying that vision happens among, or is caught in, things—in that place where something visible undertakes to see, becomes visible for itself by virtue of the sight of things; in that place where there persists . . . the undividedness of the sensing and the sensed.[3:163]

The concept of embodiment informs us that consciousness is diffused throughout the body and finds expression through it. We *are* our bodies. Bodily position in space and time, bodily movement and action shape experience by giving consciousness access to the world. There is in experience, then, a unity of the perceiving subject and the objective world. In experience there are not inner and outer realities. The inescapable relation of subject and object is what Merleau-Ponty refers to as being situated.

Merleau-Ponty discusses the phenomenon of the phantom limb to demonstrate that the experience of one's body is based on being-in-the-world:

> What it is in us which refuses mutilation and disablement is an *I* committed to a certain physical and inter-human world, who continues to tend towards his world despite handicaps and amputations and who, to this extent, does not recognize them de jure.[3:81]

Rejecting physiological and psychological explanations as inadequate, Merleau-Ponty acknowledges that the phantom limb can be related to both. The difficulty in these explanations resides in the experience of presence of a limb that should not be given:

> The man with one leg feels the missing limb in the same way as I feel keenly the existence of a friend who is, nevertheless, not before my eyes; he has not lost it because he continues to allow for it. . . . The phantom arm is not a representation of the arm, but the ambivalent presence of an arm.[3:81]

The body as a power is assumed at a preobjective level, and the amputated limb, a customary part of this being. The person with a phantom limb is living his body in the way to which he is accustomed.

This phenomenological view of the phantom limb is not a denial of physiological facts or of psychological explanations of memory, belief or acceptance. Rather, it introduces a common ground for these facts—a situation for an existence. The unity of the human organism can be understood only at this level of preobjective experience.

In Schutz's discussion of attention to life, he describes our interest in life as variable and as seeming to vary by levels of tension. The plane of action in the world is the highest level of tension as it represents our highest interest in meeting reality and its requirements. Action in the world is a fully directed involvement with the world. Schutz refers to this active engagement in present experiences as wide-awakeness. At this level, the person is committed to carrying through his intentions in the world.[5:68-69] The patient with a phantom limb might try, for example, to reach for something with his amputated arm. In his lived body and in his attention to action, the reach makes perfect sense and is not simply a matter of psychological denial or physiological nerve transmission extension. It is only as this engagement with the world in action is suspended that the patient can consider the truth of the amputated limb and compensate for a lived body that may continue to press toward the world for some time.

The phantom limb is a transient phenomenon. The patient's perception ultimately is replaced with another perception from the new perspective given through his body. The amputated limb gives rise to experiences that pass through time to direct his attention to life in new ways. This is not accomplished by thinking about it but, rather, by living it through time.

EXPERIENCE AND PERCEPTION

Merleau-Ponty explains that the inherence of one's body in the world forms a system. Life experience is mediated through bodily experience of lived correspondence among objects. Meanings are possible only as one takes up a position in space.

> If there is, for me, a cube with six equal sides, and if I can link up with the object, this is not because I constitute it from the inside: It is because I delve into the thickness of the world by perceptual experience.[3:204]

> This thing, and the world, are given to me along with the parts of my body . . . in a living connection . . . identical, with that existing between the parts of my body itself.[3:105]

Living, being, experiencing, perceiving are all nothing without the world that is lived, experienced, or perceived. Lived experience is reality. Lived experience and the perceived world are terms that communicate the indivisible experiencing subject and experienced object.

Lived experience is the focus of attention in phenomenology rather than the process of experiencing. Just as consciousness is indistinct from the world toward which it is directed, the act of perceiving is inextricable from the perceived world.

> I am not a "living being" or even a "man" or even a "consciousness" with all the characteristics which zoology, social anatomy or inductive psychology attributes to these products of nature or history. I am the absolute source. My ex-

istence does not come from my antecedents or my physical and social entourage, but rather does toward them and sustains them. For it is I that make exist for myself (and hence "be" in the only sense that the word can have for me) that tradition which I choose to adopt or that horizon whose distance from me tends to disappear, since it would have no such property as distance were I not there to view it.[2:60]

It is important to stress again that the world is always there for the phenomenologist. It is an inexhaustible reservoir from which reality is drawn. It is not created by the subject's involvement with it, but it is discovered through perception.

For Merleau-Ponty the world is not perceived through a combination of sensations and perspectives. Reality is not constituted by perceiving representations of reality. Coherence in the world is lived. Relation with the world is a living impulse, irreducible, and understandable only as unified experience. It is not knowledge of the world such as is posed by an analysis of sensation.

Perception is defined as access to truth—the foundation of all knowledge. Having established being-in-the-world as embodied consciousness constituting experience, perception refers to the original awareness of that engagement of human life in the world. Perception gives one access to experience of the world as it is given prior to any analysis of it: "To perceive is to render oneself present to something through the body. All the while the thing keeps its place within the horizon of the world."[3:42] The world as perceived is the first reality.

Perception, in Merleau-Ponty's view, is distinguished from the scientific explanation of it as an act of consciousness, in the same way that deciding and reasoning are acts of consciousness. Perception cannot be understood through an analysis of sensation as an object.

Merleau-Ponty's description of perception begins with the explanation that perception does not depend on external stimuli as if they were clear, defined, unambiguous. Rather, stimuli are perceived in the context of the experience to which they belong:

> To see is to have colours or lights, to hear is to have sounds, to sense is to have qualities. . . . But red and green are not sensations, they are the sensed, and quality is not an element of consciousness, but a property of the object. Instead of providing a simple means of delimiting sensations, if we

consider it in the experience itself which evinces it the quality is as rich and mysterious as the object, or indeed the whole spectacle, perceived.[3:4]

To clarify these statements, Merleau-Ponty explains that seeing a red patch on a carpet is contingent on shadows and lights, size, and the wool fabric of the carpet. This red would not be the same in the absence of these "meanings which reside in it." It is not possible to perceive sensations, like the color red, without the overlays that form experience. What Merleau-Ponty attempts to establish with this argument is the error in presuming that there is something reliable and constant in sensation of objective stimuli. Perception is awareness of the appearances of phenomena, and it must see the red patch on the carpet as it really is, with shadow, light, size, and wool. From this totality, one is able to conceive of this particular red.

Perception is the original mode of consciousness. Whereas the body gives us access to the world, perception is our access to experience in the world, as it is presented to us before reflection. We perceive through our bodies. Bodily being-in-the-world is the field and home of experience and perception.

The perceived world is a unified one in which relations are comprised and organized. Merleau-Ponty refers to this as a practical synthesis, distinguished from a conceptual or intellectual one. The perceived world is a totality open to an infinite variety of perspectives, merging in a unique, individual style, to define one's reality. Merleau-Ponty's discussion of perceiving a specific object—a lamp—elucidates this phenomenological theme:

I grasp the unseen side as present, and I do not affirm that the back of the lamp exists in the same sense that I say a solution of a problem exists. The hidden side is present in its own way. It is in my vicinity.[6:14]

The perception of a lamp is of a whole lamp, a meaning prior to an intellectual process that posits the total lamp as possible or necessary, based on judgments about the reality of such an object. In perception, the lamp's reality is achieved by the subject who grasps the whole of the lamp through his perspective on one of the object's aspects. Perception, then, is not simply introspection or mere subjectivity. It is being there to see, to hear, to experience, to know. Attending to that involvement serves to bring a greater discipline to conceptions superimposed on what is learned first, in perception.

We now see that perception is the appearance of phenomena, and the perceived world is reality. This is not to be confused with truth. As access to truth, perception presents us with evidence of the world not as it is thought, but as it is lived. Perception of an amputated limb as an ambivalent presence is not truth, but it is reality. It is this evidence that is considered to be the foundation of science and knowledge. Beyond this, there is nothing to understand.

THE PHENOMENOLOGICAL METHOD

THE AIM OF PHENOMENOLOGICAL INQUIRY

The aim of phenomenology is to describe experience as it is lived by people. Human experience in a world of others, objects, events is the only consciousness that has meaning for us. The body is our access to the world, and hence the means by which experience occurs. Perception is viewed as our access to human experience. Merleau-Ponty has referred to the primacy of perception because it is the first awareness of being-in-the-world. To describe lived experience, then, we are directed to the perceived world. Reflective thought is used in the effort to grasp or to understand the meaning of what one is living through. The data examined in reflection are that of being-in-the-world, not of an interior set of facts. The distinction presented earlier between reality and truth is emphasized in delineating the focus of study. It is the experience, for example, of loving and doubting, or of the phantom limb, that calls for description in phenomenology; not an analysis of what love is, or an explanation of what causes the phantom limb to appear.

Phenomenology is an approach that concentrates on the subject's experience rather than concentrating solely on subjects or on objects. For example, the focus in phenomenology would be on the client's perception of being hospitalized rather than a focus on roles, the family system, health care technology, and so on, in piecemeal fashion. The focus in phenomenology enlarges our view by attempting to "see" human experience in the complexity of its context. The effort in phenomenology to disclose human experience is a concern with giving phenomena a fuller and fairer hearing than empiricism accords them.

PHENOMENOLOGICAL REDUCTION AND DESCRIPTION

In phenomenological description, analysis and explanation are pointedly excluded, whether it be from a philosophically minded introspection or a rigorous scientific framework. Schutz's comments on man as being biographically determined call attention to the difficulty in making these exclusions:

> Man finds himself at any moment of his daily life in a biographically determined situation, that is, in a physical and sociocultural environment as defined by him, within which he has his position, not merely his position in terms of physical space and outer time or of his status and role within the social system but also his moral and ideological positions.[5:73]

This is to say that one's lived experience is always determined by one's history, and by what Schutz refers to as "the sedimentation of all man's previous experiences." These are part of the person and world in their relation, and are hence enmeshed in experience.

Lived experience is in this sense layered with meanings that are brought to the relation of being-in-the-world. One way this occurs is through the selection of attention to life. In Merleau-Ponty's explanation, this corresponds with the idea of taking up a perspective in the world, whereby a horizon and a figure-ground relation appears.

The objective in phenomenological description is, nevertheless, to forage through these layers to rediscover the first experience, before we use our knowledge and beliefs to make a new sense out of experience. The gain in this effort resides in a closer adherence between knowledges and the experiences to which they refer.

The perceived world is at each moment filled with stimuli and presences that are not precisely connected in a contextual framework. They are, however, unhesitatingly recognized as belonging to the world and being real. Phenomena in the perceived world are related without judgment or other acts of consciousness such as expecting, believing, knowing. It is on the foundation of perception, the original awareness, that all such acts are constructed. The real, lived experience is given in the perceived world; and this is what must be described.

How to recognize lived experience, as it is presented in perception, is the final and most difficult phenomenological theme to be presented here. Merleau-Ponty describes the scope of this task.

> Our relation to the world is so profound and so intimate that the only way for us to notice it is to suspend its movements, to refuse it our complicity . . . or to render it inoperative.[2:64]

He instructs us to make our presuppositions and common sense appear by deliberately abstaining from them. He advises us to be astonished before the world. In other words, in order to describe lived experience, we must set aside the natural attitude toward the world that our biography gives us. In astonishment, the layers of meaning given by interpretation, knowledge, and explanation are carefully preserved but laid aside. Our ties to the world in roles, knowledge, belief, habit, common sense, and the like, are disrupted in order to make them apparent. Bracketing our presuppositions about the world is performed "not to deny them and even less to deny the link which binds us to the physical, social and cultural world."[6:49]

The process of recovering original awareness is called "reduction" in phenomenology. Complete reduction is impossible because consciousness is engaged in a world. Phenomenological description is always contingent, then, on the perspective given in experience and presented in perception. Further, in the reflection of reduction, which strives to freeze time and suspend acts of consciousness, time nevertheless continues. There is always in phenomenological description, then, the layer of this experience in time, in the study of the experience that has just passed: "Our existence is too strictly caught up in the world to know itself as such at the moment when it is thrown forth upon the world."[2:65] For this reason, phenomenological reduction and description will yield incomplete profiles of reality, because one can never surpass time.

Schutz's attempt to eliminate the mysteriousness that tends to surround phenomenological method assists in illuminating the complex idea of reduction. He starts by acknowledging that the technique of bracketing in reduction is extremely difficult but yet within human capability. In performing the reduction, one assumes an attitude of doubt toward the world.

> What we have to put in brackets is not only the existence of an outer world, along with all the things in it, inanimate

and animate, including fellow-men, cultural objects, society and its institutions. Also our belief in the validity of our statements about this world and its content, as conceived within the mundane sphere, has to be suspended. Consequently, not only our practical knowledge of the world but also the propositions of all the sciences dealing with the existence of the world, all natural and social sciences, psychology, logic and even geometry—all have to be brought within the brackets.[4:105]

As the layers of meaning that give us interpreted experience are laid aside, what remains is the perceived world. In the perceived world, objects appear in a figure-ground relation. Each object has a horizon implicating other objects. In the perceived world, objects, events, people are not experienced in isolation. Instead, they are presented in perception in a meaningful system of relations. This is the meaning of holism; and perception is the level at which holism occurs.

As Schutz states, "we just make up our mind to refrain from any judgment concerning spatiotemporal existence" in order to reveal perception.[5:58] While this explanation of the phenomenological reduction succeeds in demysticizing this technique in the method, it should not be construed to mean that this is a simple matter. One has only to attempt to suspend the common-sense natural attitude toward the world to appreciate the conditions necessary for such a task. Long periods of undisturbed time are not the least of these; and, in the context of most occupational demands, such conditions simply do not exist for most of us. This makes Schutz's description of the natural attitude as a constitution of layers of meaning useful in a consideration of reduction as a method that can be used in degrees. Layers can be peeled away one at a time. Perception can be revealed relatively to such a painstaking effort to peel away some of our ready-made interpretations of experience.

Our knowledge of an object, at a certain given moment, is nothing else than the sediment of previous mental processes by which it has been constituted. It has its own history, and this history of its constitution can be found by questioning it. This is done by turning back from the seemingly ready-made object of our thought to the different activities of our mind in which and by which it has been constituted step by step.[4:111]

In a simplified sense, reduction is being used whenever one turns toward one's experience in a reflective mood that questions the knowledge one has of one's experience.

The outcome of reduction, the world that remains after bracketing, are the appearances of phenomena as they are given in perception, prior to interpretation and explanation. Schutz explains the usefulness of such efforts:

> Since to each empirical determination within the phenomenological reduction there necessarily corresponds a parallel feature within the natural sphere and vice versa, we can always turn back to the natural attitude and there make use of all the insights we have won within the reduced sphere.[5:59]

This outcome of enrichment in the world of knowledge needs to be emphasized and distinctly contrasted with a misunderstanding of phenomenology as an alternative in a stream of choices in knowing.

ESSENTIAL STEPS AND OPERATIONS

Spiegelberg has described the essentials of phenomenological method in the belief that these constitute the characteristic core in the various phenomenologies. Although identifying and eliminating the assumptions with which we see the world is acknowledged as a difficult task, Spiegelberg regards "the emancipation from preconceptions" as the primary tangible contribution of phenomenology and its most teachable part.[1:656–57]

In a discussion of seven steps of phenomenological method, Spiegelberg states that the first three steps are accepted and practiced by those who align themselves with the phenomenological movement; the last four steps, by a smaller group. For this reason, the first three steps will be described here as a general framework for the various interpretations of phenomenological method that can be found in the literature. These steps are:

1. Investigating particular phenomena.
2. Investigating general essences.
3. Apprehending essential relationships among essences.

Spiegelberg notes that the first of these steps, investigating particular phenomena, is easily the most adoptable and has a completeness of its own. Because this step is viewed as primary in its applicability to nursing research, this description focuses on it. Steps 2 and 3 are then described in less detail. The interested reader is referred to Spiegelberg's discussion for a complete description of these as well as the more controversial steps in phenomenological method.[1:656-57]

Within step 1, the first operation is to intuit the phenomena:

It is one of the most demanding operations, which requires utter concentration on the object intuited without becoming absorbed in it to the point of no longer looking critically. Nevertheless there is little that the beginning phenomenologist can be given by way of precise instructions beyond such metaphoric phrases as "opening his eyes," "keeping them open," "not getting blinded," "looking and listening," etc.[1:659-60]

Comparing and contrasting the phenomenon under investigation with related phenomena, and studying phenomenologists' approaches to and accounts of phenomena are also offered as aids in learning to perform this operation.

The second operation, phenomenological analyzing, involves identifying the structure of the phenomena according to their ingredients and their configuration. As the phenomenon is distinguished with regard to its elements or constituents, its relations to and connections with adjacent phenomena are also explored.

The third and last operation, phenomenological describing, is undertaken after phenomenological "seeing" in intuiting and analyzing the phenomena has been accomplished:

Phenomenology begins in silence. Only he who has experienced genuine perplexity and frustration in the face of the phenomena when trying to find the proper description for them knows what phenomenological seeing really means.[1:672]

Spiegelberg cautions that premature description is, in fact, one of the main pitfalls of phenomenology. The aim of this describing operation is to communicate: to guide the listener by giving distinctive "guideposts" to the phenomena. The description serves to direct the listener to his own experience of the phenomena, actual or potential.

Describing is based on a classification of the phenomena. A description, therefore, presupposes a framework of class names, and all it can do is to determine the location of the phenomenon with regard to an already developed system of classes.[1:673]

In the case of new phenomena or new aspects of familiar phenomena, there will not be any such existent framework to house the description. Then, Spiegelberg advises, description of negation, metaphor, and analogy can be used cautiously to indicate the phenomena in a suggestive manner. Phenomenological description is always necessarily selective, and as such poses another major pitfall. Rather than concentrating on the central characteristics of the phenomenon, tangents and irrelevancies might be focused on.

The second step of the phenomenological method described by Spiegelberg as implicit to the various phenomenologies is investigating general essences. Based on antecedent or simultaneous intuiting of particulars, given in perception or in imagination, this step involves looking at the particulars as examples or instances that represent the general essence. For example, focusing on the particular sarcastic statement of an individual, we can understand it as an instance of sarcasm in general. This particular sarcastic comment exemplifies sarcasm and, finally, anger as such. Use of this step requires looking through particular instances to apprehend their natural affinity. The search for general essence is a search for a common pattern shared by particular phenomena that belong together in a natural grouping. "Thus what happens is that on the basis of seeing particulars in their structural affinities we also become aware of the ground of their affinities, the pattern or essence."[1:678] The same operations of analysis and description in the first step of phenomenological method described above would then be used.

The third and last step to be considered here is apprehending essential relationships. The aim in this step is to discover essential relationships or connections pertaining to essences apprehended in the second step. These essential relationships may be within a single essence or between several essences. Spiegelberg notes that the adverb "essentially" usually points to such relationships.

An operation of free imaginative variation of omission or substitution is used to determine if the components of an essence are or are not essential to it. For example, in the case of the essence "rapport," the phenomenologist would consider whether or not rapport remains an essence without the essential elements of trust and respect, or whether or not rapport remains an essence by replacing these elements with others, such as dependency and authority.

Imaginative variation is also used to apprehend essential relationships between essences:

> Keeping one essence constant we try to combine it with various other essences, leaving off some of its associates, substituting others for them, or adding essences not hitherto encountered together with them. . . . The question at issue is whether or not several essences stand in relationships not contained in either of them alone, but entailed by them jointly.[1:682]

Through imaginative variation, the phenomenologist uses experience and intuitive procedures in conjunction to synthesize knowledge about a phenomenon.

Phenomenological analysis clarifies phenomena by "replacing habitual concepts, to which we pay no careful attention, by concepts which are consciously clarified and are therefore far less likely to remove us from experience as it is lived."[6:61] In performing the reduction, one suspends one's preconceptions in order to explore the phenomenon not from what is known about it, but from what might be so. Merleau-Ponty refers to this process and "the imaginary 'free variation' of certain facts":

> In order to grasp an essence, we consider a concrete experience, and then we make it change in our thought, trying to imagine it as effectively modified in all respects. That which remains invariable through these changes is the essence of the phenomena in question.[6:70]

This is fundamentally the same mode as that of induction when it moves toward constructing concepts that describe common elements among cases. "You link together the different examples effectively perceived by an imaginary variation which will lead from one to the other."[6:7]

Merleau-Ponty points out that the difference between induction and phenomenological reduction and description is a matter of degree. In this sense, science and phenomenology converge, rather than complement or supplant each other.

INTERPRETATIONS OF THE METHOD

Omery reports that the multiple interpretations and modifications of phenomenology can be attributed to the fact that, as a movement, phenomenology remains in a process of clarification.[7:50] In the United States phenomenology has not flourished, although one can identify and trace a following in sociology and psychology. In these disciplines, phenomenological method has been interpreted in a somewhat definitive manner in a sequence of procedural steps. Omery notes that the development of definitive methodology is attributable to three possible causes, including an attempt to legitimate phenomenology in a scientific world that adheres to the empirical approach.[7:54–55]

A number of interpretations have been used and published, and therefore made accessible to nurses who wished to adopt phenomenological method for their studies. In Adrian Van Kaam's work, for example, phenomenological method is adapted to the study of human experience in the aim of developing a "repeatable, more or less controlled method for analyzing those modes of experiencing which seem to have general validity and are therefore useful for the construction of a lawful theory of human experience."[8:67] Based on the assumption that there is an essence in human experiences that is the same in different individuals, Van Kaam's method involves collecting descriptions of the experience under study from a large number of subjects so that it is possible to differentiate that which is constant from that which is variable from subject to subject. Written descriptions of the experience are then processed as follows: (1) exhaustive listing of every expression of the experience, (2) reduction of expressions by grouping them by labels that are faithful to the subjects' expressions, (3) elimination of expressions that do not seem to be potentially a necessary constituent of the experience, (4) continued organization of expressions into clusters that are tentatively labeled as descriptive constituents of the experience, and (5) checking the tentatively identified constituents against random cases of the sample. All these steps in analysis of the data were performed independently in Van Kaam's study of feeling as understood by three judges to ensure reliability of the results: a synthetic description of the experience with a justification and explanation of each phrase.

In Colaizzi's interpretation of phenomenological method, the method of data collection is more liberally treated to include interview, observation of the nonverbal, observation of the context, and the researcher's responses. The steps for analyzing data, once obtained, are: (1) careful study of the data in order to acquire a "feel" for them, (2) elimination of repetitive or overlapping statements in extraction of the significant, (3) formulation of meaning in each significant statement, (4) organization of statements into themes or clusters, and (5) validation of these themes with the original descriptions and final integration of the results in an exhaustive description of the phenomenon.[9]

In a nursing interpretation of phenomenological method, Paterson and Zderad describe these steps: (1) an intuitive grasp of a phenomenon that allows it to be recognized from one occasion to the next, (2) analytic examination of its occurrences, and (3) synthesis and description of the phenomenon. The intuitive grasp entails the ability to become conscious of spontaneous perceptions and to be open to the data of experience by attempting to bracket presuppositions. Alerted to the phenomenon, the researcher describes, reflects on, and questions it. Data may also be solicited from others. Techniques are described to assist the concurrent processes of analysis, synthesis, and description: (1) comparing and contrasting instances of the phenomenon to identify similarities and differences, (2) seeking characteristics or elements found in one instance of the phenomenon in others, (3) imagining the phenomenon without a particular element, (4) studying the elements to see how they are interrelated, (5) relating the phenomenon to other similar phenomena, (6) classification, if indicated, in a broader category, (7) selecting the phenomenon's central characteristics and eliminating accidentals, and (8) using negation, analogy, and metaphor to promote analysis and description.[10:83-91]

Since nurse researchers are new to phenomenology, there are few models for its use within our own discipline. With the exception of Paterson and Zderad's work, guidance in exploring this new method for nursing research has necessarily been sought from other disciplines. The pitfalls in this, however, are apparent: a research method suitable to another discipline may fail to disclose phenomena unique to the nursing world.

While we continue to learn about phenomenological method both in its essential steps and in its interpretations by others, nurse researchers need to remain unrestricted except by the fundamental themes that distinguish phenomenology as a movement. An increasingly thorough study of primary sources is therefore critical to the successful interpretation of phenomenological method. In the next section, an effort is made to extend Spiegelberg's discussion of the essential steps in phenomenological method to a description of principles and techniques guiding research design. The aim of this effort is to offer a guide to effective implementation of the method without prescribing structured procedures that might prematurely bring our exploration of the method to closure.

THE PHENOMENOLOGICAL METHOD
IN NURSING RESEARCH

In using phenomenological method in nursing research, one must adhere to certain principles, consistent with primary phenomenological themes. The first of these is the attention to subjects' realities in formulating the research question. The elusive concepts that characterize nursing concerns in practice provide the subject matter for our studies. For example, Paterson and Zderad present a study of comforting and being comforted;[10:103-129] Stanley has studied the lived experience of hope;[11] Lynch investigated the mother's experience of unplanned hospitalization of the young child;[12] Haase studied the components of courage as experienced by chronically ill adolescents;[13] and Riemen has presented her study of the essential structure of a caring interaction.[14] In each of these studies, the effort to disclose human experience in all its complexity is apparent.

Second, attention to such realities requires that the researcher approach the study with a holistic perspective. This is manifest in posing the research question generally as, for example, in Riemen's study: "From the perspectives of the client, what is the essential structure of a caring nurse–client interaction?" In addition, selection of data-collection procedures is guided by the intent to preserve the natural spontaneity of subjects' lived experiences. An effort is made to approach the research question holistically by going to people in their circumstances where they are involved in the world. In Lynch's study of unplanned hospitalization and in Paterson's study of comfort, nursing contact with clients in the clinical setting was used. For Paterson, her experiences of interacting with distressed clients was the data source; for Lynch, a research interview technique was used. For Haase and Riemen, interviews were also used, and in Haase's study interviews supplemented subjects' written descriptions. Repeated contacts with subjects to follow through with expressions is commonly introduced in the design to clarify, to validate, to exhaust the subject's expression. It may be argued that the most complete data collection procedure necessarily involves immersion in the experience through clinical involvement.

Decisions regarding data collection procedures are further influenced by a third principle: the researcher must recognize that she is herself immersed in the phenomenon of study by virtue of studying it. Because the researcher is an integral part of the research process, a range of modes of awareness can be used in data collection. The anthropological techniques of participant observation, for example, can be modified and interpreted in nursing to capitalize on the data accessible through clinical involvement with clients. Lynch used such an approach to collect data regarding the mother's experience during a child's unplanned hospitalization.

Empathic and intuitive awareness as well as the broad scope of ways in which people present their experiences to others are included in research design options. The use of the researcher's scope of awarenesses is demonstrated in the study of comfort and comforting. Relatively untapped sources of data in nursing, such as nurses' poetry[15] need to be located. Sources are limited only by our imagination and our sense of ethics.

The researcher's involvement is controlled, however, in certain ways intended to avoid idiosyncratic bias that would reduce the method to mere subjectivity in the empiricist sense. These are by: (1) explicating the researcher's perspective, (2) bracketing a priori explanation about the phenomenon, (3) selecting unfamiliar settings, people, and circumstances for the study, (4) assuming a posture of unobtrusive presence with the subjects, and (5) performing the study with a coresearcher so that dialogue can be used throughout the research process to promote transcendence of individual bias.

Phenomenology aims to describe experience rather than to define, categorize, explain, or interpret it. Enlargement, then, is the fourth principle used to guide researchers in the qualitative expression of findings. Since a successful description directs the consumer of research to his own experience of the phenomenon, actual or potential, the tests of validity reside in the consumer. Are the findings recognized to be true by those who live the experience? If the consumer's experience is potential, can the experience be recognized after reading (or seeing or listening to) the description of it? If the experience is skill-oriented, such as reassuring another, does the study enable the reader to live that experience?[16]

Communication of phenomenological findings need not be restricted to narrative descriptions. Photographs[17] and poems are examples of options. In order to relate phenomenological findings to the world of existing theory, a review of the literature may be performed after the data are in. Theory used to assist with communicating findings should be carefully explicated and monitored so that the insights gained into the phenomena are not lost.

ESTABLISHING A PHENOMENOLOGICAL BASELINE IN NURSING RESEARCH

The phenomenological baseline in nursing is the "real" world of living and experiencing of the patient, family, and nurse. In nursing research and theory, it is a thorough description of our nursing world as it is experienced by the participants. A phenomenological baseline, when established, would provide fully developed nursing concepts that are faithful to the real world of lived nursing experience. With these clarified concepts of the nursing world, nursing theory and empirical studies deduced from our theories would possess a greater relevance in their comments about nursing since they would adhere more closely to nursing realities. Establishing a phenomenological baseline —a coherent and accurate description of lived experience—will be accomplished through qualitative studies. The process is one of theory development, and empirical studies are examples of second-order comment. A few examples may clarify these points.

Phenomenology directs us to study human experience with a serious effort to reconsider foundations in our views that lead us to conceptualized, interpreted experience rather than a clear view of what we live through. Nursing management of dependency in the nursing situation, for example, may suffer from a lack of such attention to the meanings of dependency in various nursing situations. Consider, for example, how being bathed might facilitate recovery through a mechanism such as therapeutic touch. Or how uncontrolled diabetes facilitates another goal by maintaining the noncompliant diabetic patient's relationship with a visiting nurse. Or how ministering to clients makes it possible for nurses to be emotionally available to them.

In this example of dependency, the phenomenological base-line for practice and research would provide a thorough descrip-tion of human dependency in nursing situations. We would ask, "Dependent upon whom, for what, with what consequences, what are the alternatives, and how does being dependent 'figure in' with one's health, with striving toward and achieving one's goals in one's world?" The baseline would provide us with a clarified concept of dependency. This would be a nursing concept; one that might vary from the perspective and the truth in psychology or in sociology. On the other hand, when thoroughly described, a nursing concept of dependency might be instructive to other disciplines.

A second example of ways in which phenomenology might be used to advance nursing science concerns access to client experience. As many prominent nurse scholars have pointed out, much of what makes nursing unique is grounded in our presence in people's lives when they are in crisis, as during illness and hospitalization, and when the nurse is the most qualified health professional available, as in some community-based practices. Identifying oneself as a nurse is nearly always sufficient to gain entry into a client's situation. Often, this is expressed in a one-way physical intimacy with amazingly minimal embarrassment or shame for the client.

Nurses' ready access to clients' experiences enables nurses to assess and to render assistance quickly. Further, the duration of nursing care over time—both hour-to-hour mundane living time and day-to-day, month-to-month time in illness and recovery—is a unique feature of nursing service. This temporal characteristic of nursing gives us access to clients' experiences through a special kind of involvement in their lives. And the yield is a quantitatively and qualitatively different kind of data than that obtained from a client's best attempt to describe his situation in a focused interview, for example, or his best attempt to present his situation on a questionnaire.

Sally Gadow has described the wealth of different kinds of data that a nurse and client have access to and can use in the client's interest. These include the nurse's empathic and sym-pathetic, aesthetic and ethical, as well as scientific and objective awarenesses, for example.[18] Attending a client through a night when he has pain and cannot sleep clearly has the potential of yielding different and infinitely richer data than an hour's as-sessment of the client's pain using customary measures. In this unique access to human experience, the nursing practitioner is also in a unique position to perform research. The case study in particular is too infrequently exploited for the understandings it can give us of human experience as well as of the efficacy of nursing interventions.

Alternatively, as an outsider, the nurse researcher might create a design resembling a montage, a collection of data-gathering techniques with an *N* of one or two to accomplish a case study. This montage might include participant observation with the researcher engaging in giving care at times, but flexibly so. It might include interview techniques as well as discrete observations; recorded data as well as solicited data.

In selecting data-collecting techniques and strategies, the researcher has a broader range of choices when she strives to become enmeshed in the situation as thoroughly as possible and yet maintain the researcher role. This is consistent, phenomenologically, with the idea that the person is inevitably enmeshed in the world around him. It is also faithful to the phenomenological prescriptive to be generous in allowing phenomena to speak fully.

The aim of phenomenology, again, is to describe lived experience. And we accomplish this through attention to the perceived world, to the question of how phenomena appear to people in experience. The subject matter of phenomenological inquiry is thus such experience as being in pain, doubting treatment, hoping to be well again, recovering, or preparing for discharge. These are not interior, subjective states, but rather references to living through engagement with the world. The experiential unit selected for attention may be large or small, but in every case these engagements are enormously complex.

Being in pain, for example, is an experience constituted on one's biography as well as on current stimuli and presences. Believing that one's pain is an unjust punishment, or knowing that it is caused by obstructed blood flow to the organ, are examples of information *about* pain that one uses to interpret experience. Such secondary sense-making of experience is often automatic.

The meanings of many concepts in nursing need to be carefully questioned. Dependency, self-care, patient, client, autonomy, and health, for example, are all concepts that would usefully be clarified not by a logical deduction from what is already known about them but by an exploratory process of what might be so.

Lifting the layers of interpretation from such experiencing as being dependent, healthy, or autonomous requires knowing what we know, and thinking what we do. This is to say that we become more aware of our knowledge about dependent behavior when we deliberately doubt it. And this places us in the position of being able to choose to think about dependency differently; to choose to be with dependent patients differently. In essence, we are able to choose our experiences to an extent.

Performing the reduction in nursing will mean coming to a fuller awareness of assumptions about people, health, and helping; a fuller awareness of the interpretations of experience that are both automatic and deliberate in nursing. The phenomenological perspective would lead us to think again about what is real in the experience that just passed. We would hold our knowledge in doubt; we would think again and perhaps come to a richer understanding about our clients, ourselves, and how to assist. Such understandings are directly related to the development of a body of knowledge and the design of effective nursing care. To contribute to a body of knowledge, these understandings must be described. Phenomenological description is simply the effective communication of insights into human experience.

Ours is a relatively unexamined world; establishing a phenomenological baseline in nursing would elevate this unexamined life to a new level of understanding and appreciation. The product of efforts to focus and to describe nursing phenomena in rich detail will be a mature nursing identity capable of stimulating and guiding empirical studies in our discipline. The enhanced relevance in empirical comments about nursing from such studies will in turn serve to diminish our problems with recruiting and retaining nurse researchers and with promoting utilization of research findings. Lastly, qualitative studies that yield descriptions of lived nursing experience are also ends in themselves: sources of vicarious experience, opportunity for dialogue and validation, and inspiration for practice.

NOTES

1. H. Spiegelberg, *The Phenomenological Movement*, Vols. I and II (The Hague: Martinus Nijhoff, 1976).
2. M. Merleau-Ponty, "What is Phenomenology?" *Cross Currents*, 6 (1956): 59–70.

3. M. Merleau-Ponty, *Phenomenology of Perception*, C. Smith, trans. (New York: Humanities Press, 1962).
4. A. Schutz, *Collected Papers I: The Problem of Social Reality* (The Hague: Martinus Nijhoff, 1973).
5. A. Schutz, *On Phenomenology and Social Relations* (Chicago: University of Chicago Press, 1970).
6. M. Merleau-Ponty, *The Primacy of Perception*, J. Edie, trans. (Evanston: Northwestern University Press, 1964).
7. A. Omery, "Phenomenology: A Method for Nursing Research," *Advances in Nursing Science*, 5 (1983): 49–63.
8. A. Van Kaam, "Phenomenal Analysis: Exemplified by a Study of the Experience of 'Really Feeling Understood,' " *Journal of Individual Psychology*, 15 (1959): 66–72.
9. P. Colaizzi, "Psychological Research as the Phenomenologist Views It," in R. Vaile and M. King, *Existential Phenomenological Alternatives for Psychology* (New York: Oxford University Press, 1978).
10. J. Paterson and L. Zderad, *Humanistic Nursing* (New York: John Wiley & Sons, 1976).
11. T. Stanley, *The Lived Experience of Hope: The Isolation of Discrete Descriptive Elements Common to the Experience of Hope in Healthy Young Adults*, unpublished doctoral dissertation, Catholic University of America, Washington, D.C., 1978.
12. M. M. Lynch, "Through a Mother's Eyes: The Experience of Unplanned Hospitalization of a Young Child," paper presented at the Third Annual Spring Research Symposium, Gamma Nu Chapter of Sigma Theta Tau, May 27, 1983.
13. J. Haase, "The Components of Courage: A Phenomenological Study," paper presented at American Nurses' Association Council of Nurse Researchers, Annual Meeting and Program, September 23, 1983.
14. D. Riemen, "The Essential Structure of a Caring Interaction: Doing Phenomenology," in P. Munhall and C. Oiler, *Nursing Research: A Qualitative Perspective* (Appleton-Century-Crofts, in press).
15. C. Oiler, "Nursing Reality as Reflected in Nurses' Poetry," *Perspectives in Psychiatric Care*, 21 (1983): 81–89.
16. G. Psathas, *Phenomenological Sociology: Issues and Applications* (New York: John Wiley & Sons, 1973).
17. H. Becker, "Do Photographs Tell the Truth," *Afterimage* (1978): 9–13.
18. S. Gadow, "Existential Advocacy: Philosophical Foundation of Nursing," paper presented at Phase I Conference, Four State Consortium on Nursing and the Humanities, Farmington, Connecticut, November 11, 1977.

6

CONCEPTUALIZING
HISTORICAL RESEARCH

Wanda C. Hiestand, EdD, RN
Associate Professor and Associate Director
Research Unit, Center for Nursing Research and Clinical Practice
Lienhard School of Nursing
Pace University
Pleasantville, New York

INTRODUCTION

Nursing history as an area of scholarship is still in its early stages of development. Basic descriptive studies are still uncharted in some areas. In most cases the studies are confined to narrow professional concerns. Therefore, social commentators who are using nursing history to interpret the past experience of women in this country, for example, or the professionalization of health care, must rely on incomplete, socially disconnected information. Lack of sophisticated historical knowledge about nursing calls into question our own professional self-concept and affects our public image. Far from being a single monolithic social expression, modern nursing reflects struggles, conflicts, class tensions, and territorial issues that have been played out over long periods of time. Leaving such matters unexplored by the historian denies the genuine humanity and richness of nursing's past, hampers honest analysis, and prevents us from understanding the emergence of this unique modern profession.

Invoking history is a familiar ploy for the promotion of causes or particular points of view. It is often done by selective presentation of evidence, omitting that which fails to be supportive, and biased presentation of the context of certain historical situations. Nursing history offers numerous examples of such use. The fact that nursing history has proved to be useful for interpretation of women's history, occupational history, sociological history of professionalism, as well as professional self-discovery reflects the social centrality of nurses and nursing. That some of these studies lack historical objectivity or appear to be self-serving does not make them less valuable for their insights. In a work of history, it is crucial that the genuineness of past experience be respected and presented as honestly as possible.

Developing the genuine historical context is essential and at the same time very difficult, demanding of the historiographer sensitivity to historical meaning and rigorous research efforts. Explaining the meaning of relationships in time among individual lives, as well as contemporaneous social forms and institutions and events evoked by large social forces and crises is a challenge requiring scholarly consideration from many perspectives. History is concerned with the human past and the way the present has come about; with what people have done and suffered during the course of time. The task of the historian is to present the uniqueness of yesteryear's complex human affairs and make those affairs understandable in terms of today's world. Even though history is not reproduceable because people and events are unique, we nevertheless look to history for an understanding of our world, for orientation to our present lives, and for guidance for future action.

Values, culture, and human intellect have always shaped human personality, individually and collectively. People in their social lives create and continually restructure the social forms and institutions of any society as new generations succeed the old and as larger forces and historical events create different social environments. Historical research has as its role the exploration of social change over time, "rediscovering the I in the Thou,"[1:39] in order to interpret the meaning of the past for contemporary interests and to gain understanding of human societies. This endeavor blends the humanistic and scientific traditions of scholarship.

PHILOSOPHICAL FOUNDATIONS

Traditionally, historians have placed emphasis on literary narrative to describe and discuss unique, concrete, and specific events that they believe to be significant. The critical elements by which historical research is judged remain within this tradition to a large extent. To many historians, the notion of using a "scientific" approach in history is antithetical to historical thinking. Unlike the scientist, the historian is not in search of universal laws, but rather seeks to understand the uniqueness of events and related human actions. That is to say, interpreting events with the recognition that outward expression stems from the human being's inner life as "a thought, a feeling or an act of will."[1:97]

Those are the words of Wilhelm Dilthey (1833–1911), an influential historical philosopher who wrote that all history is the rediscovery of the I in the Thou and stems from present interest. Yet individuals cannot be understood in isolation. The characteristics people share as human beings in classes, nations, or other groups can help explain the variety of people in their uniqueness and in terms of the different degrees to which individuals possess these common characteristics. Consideration of environmental factors, coupled with this quantitative approach, can help us understand individuals. Dilthey holds these beliefs as basic to understanding what he calls the mind-affected world and the interconnectedness of human life. The historian must tell a meaningful story that connects factual, concrete happenings with intangible motivations if the truth of specific events in time is to be realized. We are reminded that "the only complete, self-contained and clearly defined happening encountered anywhere in history and in every concept that occurs in human studies, is the course of a life."[1:97]

METHODOLOGICAL ISSUES AND SOCIAL HISTORY

The methodological problems of developing the historical context truthfully are well known to those who have tried to interpret or even describe the past. I have struggled with the issue of how to approach historical evidence in order to understand the emergence of modern nursing in American society.

This encompasses less than 115 years of history, fewer than six generations if a generation is counted in twenty-year periods and less than four if thirty-year periods are used.[2] Convinced that nursing history must be more broadly considered given the social importance of the nursing function, I strongly felt the need of a conceptual model in tune with current scholarship. With these thoughts in mind, and stimulated by research approaches and concepts discovered in the literature of social history and historical sociology, I set out an agenda for historical research using contemporary interpretations of the history of childhood and of the American family as an entry point for analyzing the development of modern nursing in America.[3]

The history of childhood and of the family can be categorized as part of what is often called the new social history. Social history is a fairly recent academic development difficult to define but very much in fashion and extensively discussed. E.J. Hobsbawm presents an enlightening discussion of the subject in the essay "From Social History to the History of Society," which is essentially a discussion of the potential for the uses of more objective scientific strategies for the study of historical questions emerging from the new field of social history.[4] Hobsbawm presents several definitions of the term "social history," lists some recent research subjects (as of 1971), and follows with a discussion of why models are necessary, together with some requisite characteristics of conceptual models for historical research.

Briefly, "social history" is a term used to classify the following categories of historical works:

1. It has been used to refer to the history of the poor and the lower classes, their protests and movements.
2. It refers to works difficult to otherwise classify on a variety of human activities, such as manners, customs, and everyday life: "history with the politics left out."
3. Most often, the term is associated with the historical study of economics in society stimulated by and powerfully conceptualized by Karl Marx.

Interesting and exciting questions being explored by social historians cluster around the following topics:

1. Demography and kinship.
2. Urban studies in their historical aspects.
3. Classes and social groups.
4. "Mentalities," or collective consciousness or culture.

5. Transformations of societies (industrialization or modernization).
6. Social movements and phenomena of social protest.

More recent writers would add family history and psychohistory, which encompass the history of childhood.

The remarkable worldwide growth of sociology as an academic discipline has stimulated changes in the ways of studying society so that the general historization of the social sciences has now occurred. The need for conceptual models to address historical questions related to industrialization, urbanization, and modernization seems obvious. Hobsbawm suggests that the tools and strategies effectively employed in other social sciences adapted for research of historical questions might counteract some limitations inherent in the nature of historical evidence. Methods identified as having possibilities are the statistical grouping and handling of large quantities of data, participant observation and in-depth analysis of individuals and small groups, and situations using such methods as the in-depth interview and even psychoanalytic methods. As it stands, without these newer techniques for discovery, the older historical methods scarcely permit advances "beyond a combination of the suggestive hypothesis and the apt anecdotal illustration."[4:27]

No matter which scientific disciplinary model is used for historical analysis, the special dimensions of actual events in chronological time remain as the historian's domain and starting point. Hence, a method of analysis requires "a collaboration between general models of social structure and change and the specific set of phenomena which actually occurred."[4:29] An adequate analytic model helps to broaden and deepen our understanding of American nursing and perhaps eliminate some of the confusion we face about how to interpret our professional past in terms of American society as a whole.

NURSING AND FAMILY HISTORY

I have chosen to explore nursing history from the perspective of family change, because nursing the sick and human nurture are presumed to have been central family functions throughout Western history and these functions have usually been performed by women in American society. Several contemporary writers have charged that professionalized expertise has been used as an instrument of social control by the elite over the underprivileged and that the "medicalization" of American society has subverted family self-confidence and integrity.[5-8] In more temperate language, historians agree that those American occupations that became feminized were based on women's traditional roles.[9,10]

Historians of the family have developed a large body of literature describing and analyzing the transformation of the family. The social consequences of childhood as a modern idea, the new economics of capitalism and "women's special sphere" after 1870 are explored. The broader social forces driving these social changes are conceived as urbanization, industrialization, and modernization. They are conceptualized in terms of the economic order of industrial capitalism. As modern nursing emerged as an occupation for women, some of the traditional family roles of "housekeeper, nurse of infants and the sick, educator of childhood, trainer of servants and minister of charities"[10:22] became professional roles.

The idea of family and concern for family has been a central theme throughout modern nursing, showing that the family is a key participant in health and sickness care of its members. For the first sixty years of its existence, most nursing practice took place in the home. Student nurses were explicitly prepared for private home care. Hospitals were staffed primarily by students, not by professional nurses. Nightingale's most influential book, addressed to women as health care givers in their own families, viewed health promotion and nursing as "in reality the same."[11:9]

This writing had a profound influence on American leaders such as Lillian D. Wald.[12:20] Wald was intimately involved in developing autonomous community-based nursing practice directed to the sick and the well from a consciously family-oriented perspective. Hence the work of Lillian D. Wald and public health nurses provides an entry place for exploring the historical interaction of changes in family life and professionalization of nursing. Public health nursing confronts a range of professional issues that meet at the interface of new scientific knowledge stemming from the germ theory, Darwinism, and child psychology. It deals with professionalism in itself and other allied groups and is involved in development and implementation of health-promoting social policy. Wald joined forces with other reformers of the progressive era and exercised great social leadership. Early public health nurses interacted with a clientele made up of poor immigrants and rural people. From the perspective of the dominant culture, both the newly arrived and the rurally isolated required Americanization and modern socialization. Nursing rhetoric, speaking for one part of the dominant culture, reinforced the idea of family and the unit of care, "the treatment of families in which there is sickness." Professional practice was to be centered on care of the sick with an emphasis on illness prevention and positive health. Wald wrote a series of three articles in 1904 for the *American Journal of Nursing* incorporating this comprehensive view, beginning as follows:

> The treatment of disease among the poor assumes grave importance when regarded from its social, economic and moral aspects as well as its purely therapeutic ones. . . . Interference by the State with child labor, provision for play and outdoor exercise, and vigilant inspection of food supplies . . . are examples of general recognition of the social significance of having a well community.[13:427]

Concern for the quality of life and welfare of children in their families has been another current in nursing developed by Wald at Henry Street. Of the sick child, she wrote:

> The child in the tenement house may perhaps have unwise attention when the mother is left to herself without professional supervision, but with careful technical care from the nurse, and her wise direction of the mother's efforts that must operate to the advantage of the child.[14]

The first organized effort of the Henry Street Nurses' Settlement was to convert its backyard into a playground for healthy children and a gathering place for their parents in the evenings. The original intent when Henry Street was purchased was to use that backyard space for "cripples, chronic invalids and convalescents." By 1899 Henry Street maintained a convalescent home in Rockland County, New York, a gift of Polly Sylvan Bier. The Rest, as the convalescent home was called, moved from South Nyack to Grand-View-on-Hudson in 1903, when a large piece of property was given to Henry Street and a summer camp for girls was established as well, called Riverholm. The Rest was built for nine patients and a trained nurse in attendance. It was open all year, and admission was not dependent on a physician's order, but based on the public health nurse's judgment.

Several summer vacation places were maintained by Henry Street as a response to the dismal lives led by children of the Lower East Side of Manhattan. Inadequate sanitation, vermin, crowding, poor diet, and poor health care led to an inevitable result—uncontrolled communicable disease. Slum dwellers were regularly ravaged by epidemics made worse by a depressed economy. Many children worked long hours for low wages and assumed family burdens beyond their years. Often mothering in a family was left to a child of nine or ten years. For these children, a country vacation at places like Riverholm was intended to add to personal growth through "ministrations and education." The positive effects of living in the midst of nature's beauty with good food, clean air, space for play with people who valued fun and consideration for others probably reshaped many lives. Wald believed that "good manners were minor morals." Many children were first introduced to social graces and orderly living at Riverholm by nurses. Life was lived family style in a homelike atmosphere. Riverholm was simply but attractively furnished. There were a few treasured objects, which the children learned to respect. The intimacies of life shared with nurses and other staff members allowed for the development of a relationship where guidance could be provided at critical moments as a natural part of life.[15]

There is little disagreement that professional nursing emerged from the centrality of women's sphere in family and community life experience. Historical analysis from that perspective has proved enlightening. Yet to interpret all of modern nursing history as the simple transfer of traditional feminine roles, which nurses then attempted to professionalize, fails to recognize the changing meanings of actions and the complex dynamics involved in the transformation of social attitudes.

THEORETICAL APPROACHES TO HISTORY

In developing a way to explore historical questions about the emergence of nursing as a profession, I propose some basic premises that are adapted from the writings of several historical theorists: Thomas Bender, Glen Elder, Tamara Hareven, and Lawrence Stone. Their respective areas of historical thought focus on community (Bender), the life course (Elder), delineating and differentiating the concept of time (Hareven), and collective biography, or prosopography (Stone).

To describe each briefly provides a sense of the historical questions that can then be raised. Bender proposes that community, conceived as the study of man in his wholeness rather than in roles held in a given social order, can take account of the affective human ties as well as the structural forms within which the human expressions of mutuality of sentiment took place.[16] The archetype for this view of the community is the family, both historically and symbolically.

Elder proposes a life-course model that explores the complexity of relationships among cohort groups as the dynamics of individual life proceed.[17] Interaction with life and work roles, the family unit's role in the intergenerational transmission process, and larger social forces and crises are examined. This model is deeply rooted in individual histories and careers. It places major emphasis on transitions between individual and collective behavior and social structures and roles through stages of development in time. On another level, the life-course approach demonstrates where these factors relate to the political and social aspects of historical change. This kind of research explores the interaction between life course and personality. It furthermore helps explain the causes and consequences of personality development collectively expressed, and its impact on social change.

Hareven is another prolific writer on the subject of family history.[18] Her work on time differentiation is best described by a review of her extensive bibliography. Examples of titles are, "Family Time and Industrial Time: Family and Work in a Planned Corporation Town, 1900–1924," and "Family Time and Historical Time."[18:15] To briefly summarize some of the distinctions Hareven makes: (1) "Historical time" refers to the changing social conditions reflected in linear chronological sequence, usually over decades or centuries. (2) "Family time" refers to the timing of family events within some identified sociocultural milieu that designates when family life events, roles, and transitions of individual family members take place as the family moves along its life course. (3) "Individual time" is age-related. In different societies and over time, social age may well differ from chronological age. The timing of some life events and life transitions (marriage, for example) is socially prescribed.

Stone explains the uses of "collective biography (as the modern historian calls it), multiple career-line analysis (as the social scientist calls it) or prosopography (as the ancient historians call it)."[19:46] He sees this as a valuable historical technique. "Prosopography" is defined as the investigation of the common background characteristics of a group of actors in history by means of a collective study of their lives. The idea is to establish a universe to be studied and then to ask a uniform set of questions about such matters as birth, death, marriage and family origins, social origin and inherited economic position, education, religion, occupation, and so forth. From juxtaposition and combination of such variables, significant variables are identified for internal correlations and relationship with other forms of action and behavior. Stone sees this method as a tool to attack two of the most basic problems in history, the roots of political acts and explanations of ideological or cultural changes.

This array of ideas by which to approach historical questions testifies to new excitement about history and illustrates that selection of a conceptual model is basic to sound historical analysis. With the exception of the collective biography, exemplified by *A Generation of Women: Education in the Lives of Progressive Reformers*,[20] nursing history has not been directly explored from these perspectives. Lillian D. Wald appears as one of Lagemann's reformers because Wald's leadership connects the work of nursing to the larger social arena. Wald's creation of the term "public health nursing" embodied a new concept of secularization and broadening of the nursing function, a concept hailed as the most important development of the public health movement.[21]

FEMININE EXPERIENCE OF PROFESSIONALIZATION

The roots of professionalization for nursing spring from female experience and hence have a very different social context from medicine and other male-dominated professions. Recent historical analysis emphasizes professionalizing impulses rooted in masculine experiences with elitism, power, and social control through political dominance.[22] While both men and women experienced a relation to elitism, power, social control, and political dominance, the nature of that experience was defined by gender and was qualitatively different. Historical exploration of women's experience clearly raises the issue of how professionalization proceeded in female-dominated occupations. If ties of mutuality and sentiment can define the experience of community, then historical questions can be asked as to what structural forms contained the experience of community in American history as well as what relationships existed between the identified community and the political and economic institutions at various points in time.[16:10]

Furthermore, the American experience is unique with respect to the rise of professions. Americans came to be dominated by work, identifying themselves more with their occupations than with family, religion, or community, thus creating a social structure different from that in European societies. Professionalization provided a new way to allocate wealth and social power based on individual merit rather than inheritance.[22] This suggests a transitive connection between the strong concern with family in nursing and identification of hospital and community-based groups of nurses as "the family." If a dominant self-perception of nurses as a family or community (in Bender's sense) of women indeed provided the frame of reference for nursing practice and organization, then the focus on extending the affective qualities of mutuality and sentiment outward to others provides a different logic for how professional development proceeded from that of, for example, the medical profession. Family and community are essentially similar concepts from this perspective, and so a conceptual model embodying the dimensions of individual life course, family cycle, and career and role transitions for personality development and historical timing is appropriate.

Combining Bender's idea of family as community, Stone's generational categories, the life-course model of Elder, and Hareven's ideas of time has assisted me in systematizing the masses of historical evidence and data in developing historical questions. Attempts to place individuals within time parameters based on date of birth in order to develop cohort groups and generational identification proved to be arbitrary and were rejected in frustration. Discovery of the dynamic and multileveled approach developed by Elder may, with some variation, accommodate well to nursing history. My own use of these ideas has been to accept the implied self-perception of early nurse leaders as a family and thus to think of nurses as an occupational family with all the complex sharing and interpersonal tensions implied. If the profession is the family, then nurses entering, developing, and interacting with each other and with the world at large can be perceived in a developmental way through time. Given this perspective, one might study nursing leadership in terms of human relationships, in all their dimensions, as well as in terms of concrete social situations with respect to such historical issues as the development of child welfare, for example. The nurses themselves, as they become part of this occupational family, come with demographic categories that already exist as data. What kinds of families did nurses come from and have? How does nursing compare with other occupations?

Generational categories might be assigned in twenty- or thirty-year periods, as follows:

Generation	Twenty-year Period	Thirty-year Period
1	1873–1893	1873–1903
2	1893–1913	1903–1933
3	1913–1933	1933–1963
4	1933–1953	1963–1993
5	1953–1973	
6	1973–1993	

With the development of quantitative data, individual careers might be explored in context in a more behaviorally dynamic way. Transformation of roles, patterns of experience, and meanings of nursing functions might be systematically explored, in context and intergenerationally. The specific ways an individual is both influential in and influenced by the process of historical change over time might be given stronger probability with the aid of measured variables over the life course. The timing of event, career pathway, and status levels are directly part of the life course. Personality development is seen to interact with life-course variables, and so the process of acquiring values, self-other concepts, and ego attributes can be related and perhaps better understood.

Nursing giants like Nightingale and Wald were products of their historical time. The extent to which their lives touch ours is determined by us now to the extent to which we are interested in shaping our future as nurses in American health care for the benefit of society. In the words of Dilthey, "thus the present is filled with the past and carries the future within itself."[1:105]

NOTES

1. W. Dilthey, *Pattern and Meaning in History: Thoughts on History and Society,* H. P. Rickman, ed. (New York: Harper Paperback, 1962).
2. *Daedalus: Generation,* 4 (Fall 1978), entire issue.
3. W. Hiestand, "Nursing, the Family, and the 'New' Social History," *Advances in Nursing Science,* 4 (April 1982): 1–12.
4. E. J. Hobsbawm, "From Social History to the History of Society," *Daedalus: Historical Studies Today,* 100 (Winter 1971): 20–45.
5. C. Lasch, *Haven in a Heartless World: The Family Besieged* (New York, Basic Books, 1979).
6. C. Lasch, "Life in the Therapeutic State," *New York Review of Books,* June 12, 1980, pp. 24–32.
7. B. Ehrenreich and D. English, *For Her Own Good: 150 Years of Experts' Advice to Women* (Garden City, New York: Anchor Press/Doubleday, 1978).
8. M. S. Larson, *The Rise of Professionalism: A Sociological Analysis* (Berkeley: University of California Press, 1977).
9. C. N. Degler, *At Odds: Women and the Family in America from the Revolution to the Present* (New York: Oxford University Press, 1980).
10. S. Rothman, *Women's Proper Place: A History of Changing Ideals and Practices 1870 to the Present* (New York: Basic Books, 1978).
11. F. Nightingale, *Notes on Nursing: What It Is and What It Is Not* (New York: Appleton-Century, 1938).
12. B. Siegel, *Lillian Wald of Henry Street* (New York: Macmillan, 1983).
13. L. D. Wald, "The Treatment of Families in Which There is Sickness," *American Journal of Nursing,* 4 (1904): 427–428.
14. L. D. Wald, "The District Nurses' Contribution to the Reduction of Infant Mortality, 12 November 1909." Lillian Wald Papers, Box 34–35, Rare Books and Manuscripts Division, The New York Public Library, Astor, Lenox and Tilden Foundations.
15. L. D. Wald, *The House on Henry Street* (New York: Henry Holt and Co., 1915).
16. T. Bender, *Community and Social Change in America* (New Brunswick, New Jersey: Rutgers University Press, 1978).
17. G. Elder, "Family History and the Life Course," in T. Hareven, ed., *Transitions: The Family and the Life Course in Historical Perspective* (New York: Academic Press, 1978).
18. T. Hareven, "Introduction: The Historical Study of the Life Course," in T. Hareven, ed., *Transitions: The Family and the Life Course in Historical Perspective* (New York: Academic Press, 1978).
19. L. Stone, "Prosopography," *Daedalus: Historical Studies Today,* 100 (Winter 1971): 46–79.
20. E. C. Lagemann, *A Generation of Women: Education in the Lives of Progressive Reformers* (Cambridge, Massachusetts: Harvard University Press, 1979).
21. K. Buhler-Wilkerson, "False Dawn: The Rise and Decline of Public Health Nursing in America, 1900–1930," in E. C. Lagemann, ed., *Nursing: New Perspectives, New Possibilities* (New York: Teachers College Press, 1983).
22. J. O'Toole, "Book Review, The Culture of Professionalism: The Middle Class and Development of Higher Education in America," *Teachers College Record,* 79 (1977): 149–52.

BIBLIOGRAPHY

American Nurses' Association. *Nursing: A Social Policy Statement.* Kansas City, Mo.: American Nurses' Association, 1980.

Chinn, P. L. "Debunking Myths in Nursing Theory and Research." *Image* 17 (Spring 1985): 45–49.

Chinn, P. L., and M. K. Jacobs. *Theory and Nursing: A Systematic Approach.* St. Louis: C. V. Mosby Co., 1983.

Conway, M. E. "Toward Greater Specificity in Defining Nursing's Metaparadigm." *Advances in Nursing Science* 7 (1985): 4.

Duffey, M., and A. F. Mullenkamp. "A Framework for Theory Analysis." *Nursing Outlook* 22 (1974): 570–74.

Ehrenreich, B., and D. English. *For Her Own Good: 150 Years of Experts' Advice to Women.* Garden City, N.Y.: Anchor Press/Doubleday, 1978.

Ellis, R. "Characteristics of Significant Theories." *Nursing Research* 17 (1968): 217–22.

Fawcett, J. *Analysis and Evaluation of Conceptual Models of Nursing.* Philadelphia: F. A. Davis, 1984.

———. "The Metaparadigm of Nursing: Present Status and Future Refinements." *Image* 16 (Summer 1984): 84–87.

———. "The Relationship between Theory and Research: A Double Helix." *Advances in Nursing Science* 1 (October 1978): 49–61.

119

Feldman, H. R. "Nursing Research in the 1980s: Issues and Implications." *Advances in Nursing Science* 3 (1980): 85–92.

Flaskerud, J. H., and E. J. Halloran. "Areas of Agreement in Nursing Theory Development." *Advances in Nursing Science* 3 (Winter 1980): 1–7.

Goodwin, L., and W. Goodwin. "Qualitative vs. Quantitative Research or Qualitative and Quantitative Research?" *Nursing Research* 33 (November–December 1984): 378–80.

Gortner, S. R. "The History and Philosophy of Nursing Science and Research." *Advances in Nursing Science* 5 (January 1983): 1–8.

Hardy, M. E. "Evaluating Nursing Theory." In *Theory Development: What, Why, How?* New York: National League for Nursing, 1978.

Hiestand, W. "Nursing, the Family, and the 'New' Social History." *Advances in Nursing Science* 4 (April 1982): 1–12.

King, I. M. *A Theory for Nursing: Systems, Concepts, Process.* New York: John Wiley & Sons, 1981.

Krieger, D. *Therapeutic Touch: How to Use Your Hands to Help and Heal.* Englewood Cliffs, N.J.: Prentice Hall, 1979.

Leininger, M. M. *Qualitative Research Methods in Nursing.* Orlando, Fla.: Grune & Stratton, 1985.

Levine, M. "Adaptation and Assessment: A Rationale for Nursing Intervention." *American Journal of Nursing* 66 (1966): 2450–54.

———. The Four Conservation Principles of Nursing." *Nursing Forum* 6 (1967): 45–59.

———. *Introduction to Clinical Nursing.* 2d ed. Philadelphia: F. A. Davis, 1973.

———. "The Pursuit of Wholeness." *American Journal of Nursing,* 69 (1969): 93–98.

MacPherson, K. I. "Feminist Methods: A New Paradigm for Nursing Research." *Advances in Nursing Science* 5 (Spring 1983): 17–25.

Meleis, A. I. *Theoretical Nursing: Development and Progress.* Philadelphia: J. B. Lippincott, 1985.

Munhall, P. L. "Nursing Philosophy and Nursing Research: In Apposition or Opposition." *Nursing Research* 31 (1982): 175–77.

Munhall, P., and C. Oiler. *Nursing Research: A Qualitative Perspective.* East Norwalk, Conn.: Appleton-Century-Crofts, in press.

Newman, M. *Theory Development in Nursing.* Philadelphia: F. A. Davis, 1979.

Nightingale, F. *Notes on Nursing: What It Is and What It Is Not.* New York: Dover Publications, 1969.

Oiler, C. "Nursing Reality as Reflected in Nurses' Poetry." *Perspectives in Psychiatric Care* 21 (1983): 81–89.

———. "The Phenomenological Approach in Nursing Research." *Nursing Research* 31 (1982): 178–81.

————. "The Phenomenological Baseline in Nursing Research." Paper presented at the American Nurses' Association Council of Nurse Researchers' Annual Meeting and Program, September 21, 1983.

————. "Strategy for Theory Development: Phenomenology." Paper presented at the Second Annual Nursing Theory Conference, Boston University, March 21, 1985.

Omery, Anna. "Phenomenology: A Method for Nursing Research." *Advances in Nursing Science* 5 (1983): 49–63.

Orem, Dorothea. *Nursing: Concepts of Practice.* 2d ed. New York: McGraw-Hill Book Co., 1980.

Orlando, I. *The Discipline and Teaching of Nursing Process.* New York: Putnam, 1972.

————. *The Dynamic Nurse-Patient Relationship.* New York: Putnam, 1961.

Paterson, J. G., and L. T. Zderad. *Humanistic Nursing.* New York: John Wiley & Sons, 1976.

Quinn, J. F. "Therapeutic Touch as Energy Exchange: Testing the Theory." *Advances in Nursing Science* 6 (January 1984): 42–49.

Rogers, M. E. *An Introduction to the Theoretical Basis of Nursing.* Philadelphia: F. A. Davis, 1970.

————. "Science of Unitary Human Being: A Paradigm for Nursing." In *Family Health: A Theoretical Approach to Nursing Care*, edited by I. W. Clements and F. B. Roberts. New York: John Wiley & Sons, 1983.

————. *The Science of Unitary Man.* New York: Media for Nursing, 1980. Videotapes.

Roy, C. *Introduction to Nursing: An Adaptation Model.* 2d ed. Englewood Cliffs, N.J.: Prentice Hall, 1984.

Roy, C., and S. Roberts. *Theory Construction in Nursing: An Adaptation Model.* Englewood Cliffs, N.J.: Prentice-Hall, 1981.

Stevens, B. J. *Nursing Theory: Analysis, Application, Evaluation*, 2d ed. Boston: Little, Brown & Company, 1984.

Swanson, J. M., and W. C. Chenitz. "Why Qualitative Research in Nursing?" *Nursing Outlook* 30 (1982): 241–45.

"Testing of Nursing Theory." *Advances in Nursing Science* 6 (January 1984), entire issue.

Theory Development: What, Why, How? New York: National League for Nursing, 1978.

Thibodeau, J. A. *Nursing Models: Analysis and Evaluation.* Monterey, Calif.: Wadsworth Health Sciences Division, 1983.

Tinkle, M. B., and J. L. Beaton. "Toward a New View of Science: Implications for Nursing Research." *Advances in Nursing Science* 5 (1983): 27–36.

Travelbee, J. *Interpersonal Aspects of Nursing.* Philadelphia: F. A. Davis, 1966. 2d ed., 1971.

Walker, L. O., and K. C. Avant. *Strategies for Theory Construction in Nursing*. East Norwalk, Conn.: Appleton-Century-Crofts, 1983.

Watson, J. "Nursing's Scientific Quest." *Nursing Outlook* 30 (July 1982): 413–16.

Wiedenbach, E. "The Helping Art of Nursing." *American Journal of Nursing* 63 (1963): 54–57.

―――. "Nurses' Wisdom in Nursing Theory." *American Journal of Nursing* 70 (1970): 1057–62.

Yura, H., and G. Torres, "Today's Conceptual Frameworks within Baccalaureate Nursing Programs." In *Faculty-Curriculum Development, Part III: Conceptual Framework—Its Meaning and Function*. New York: National League for Nursing, 1975.

DATE DUE

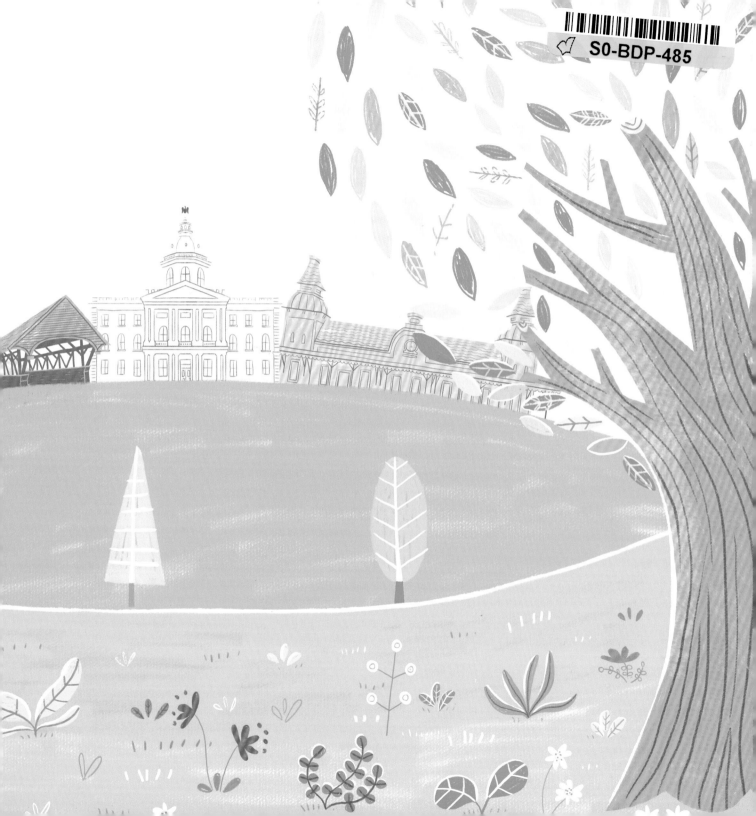

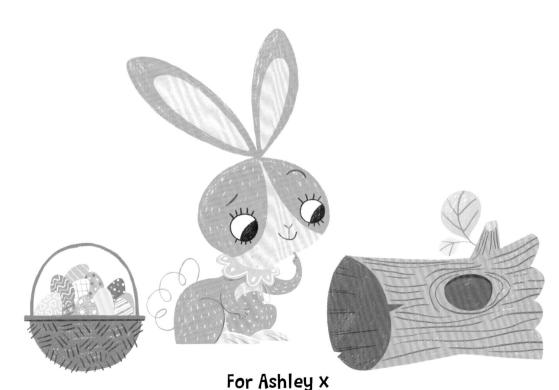

For Ashley x

Visit the author's website: www.ericjames.co.uk

Written by Eric James
Illustrated by Sara Sanchez
Designed by Nicola Moore

Published by Sourcebooks Jabberwocky, an imprint of Sourcebooks, Inc.
P.O. Box 4410, Naperville, Illinois 60567-4410
(630) 961-3900
Fax: (630) 961-2168
jabberwockykids.com

Date of Production: October 2017
Run Number: HTW_PO250717
Printed and bound in China (IMG)
10 9 8 7 6 5 4 3 2 1

Tiny the New Hampshire Easter Bunny

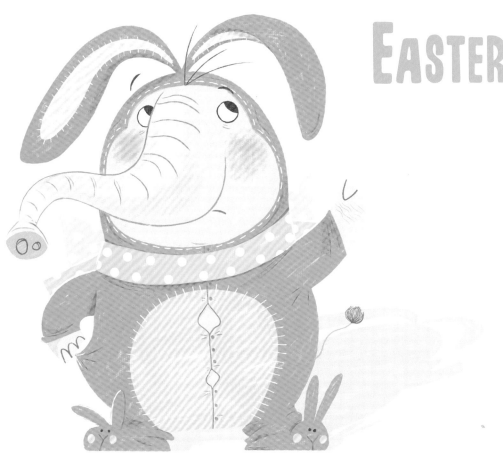

Written by
Eric James

Illustrated by
Sara Sanchez

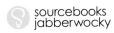
sourcebooks
jabberwocky

One bright Easter morning,
while out for a jog,

Tiny hears,

"**HELP!**
I AM STUCK
IN A LOG."

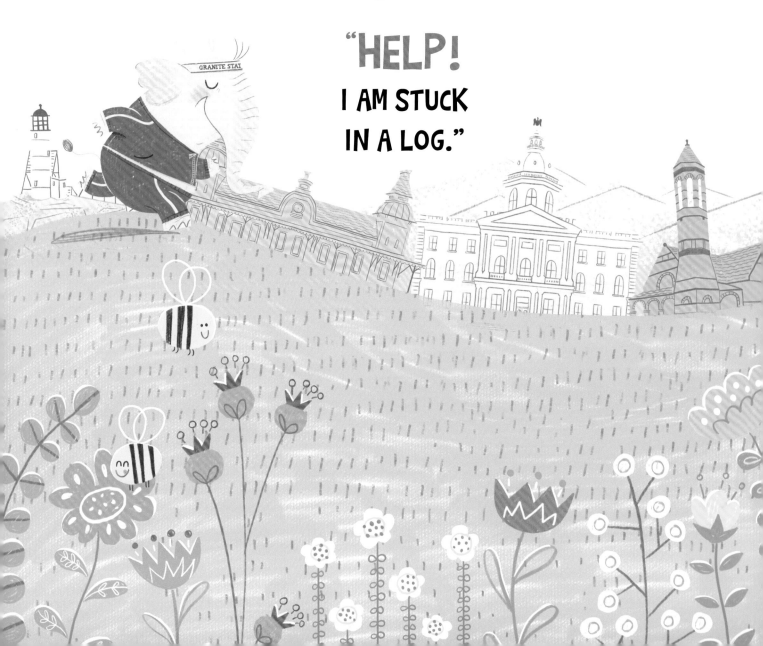

He scratches his head,
thinking, "Who could that be?
It sounded like Fluff!
I had better go see."

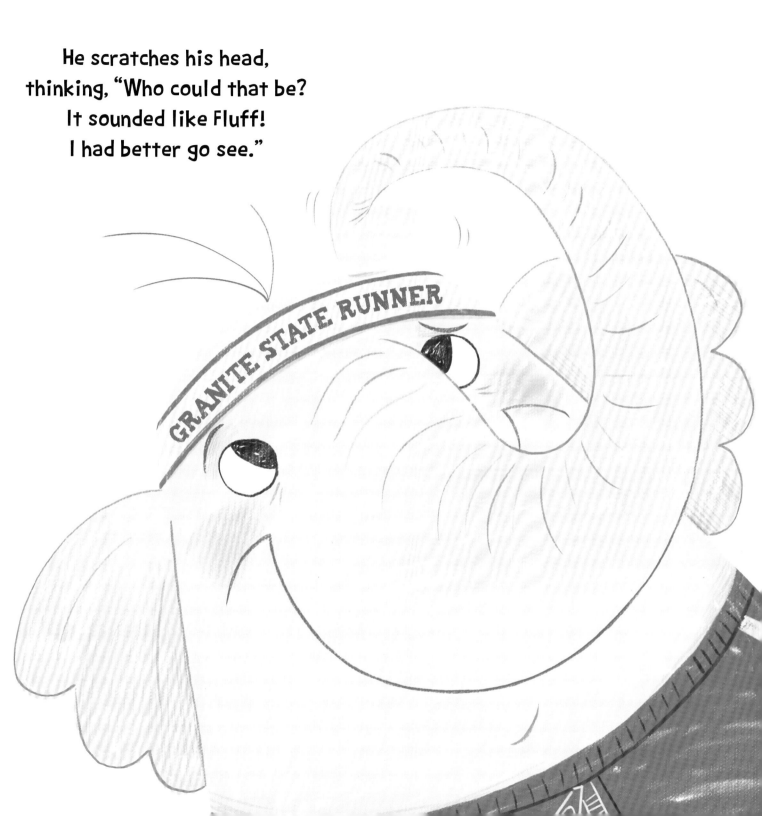

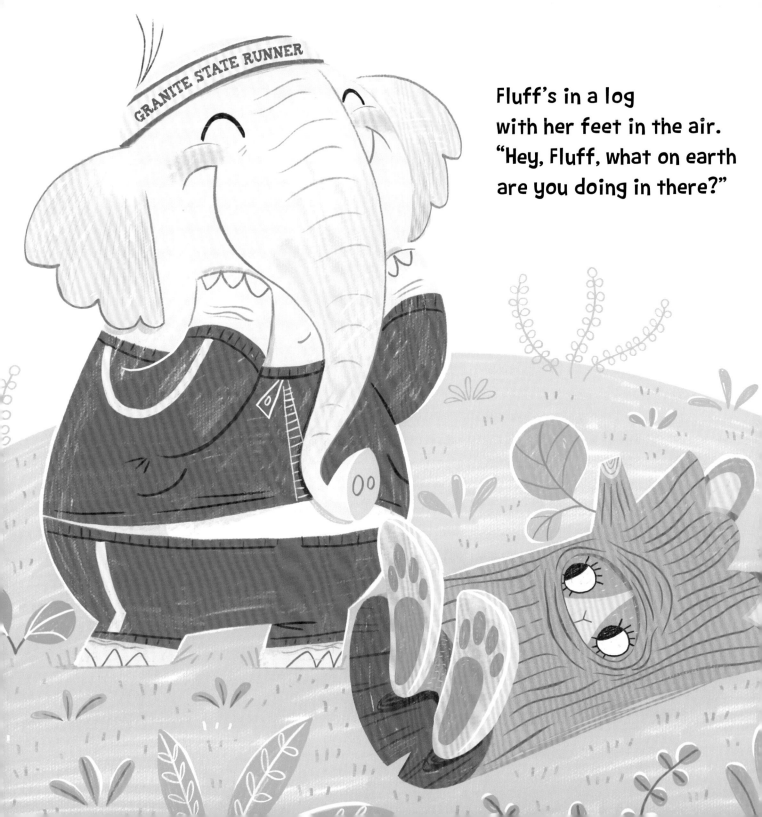

Fluff's in a log
with her feet in the air.
"Hey, Fluff, what on earth
are you doing in there?"

A sad little voice
from an echoey space
says, "I thought this would make
a good egg-hiding place."

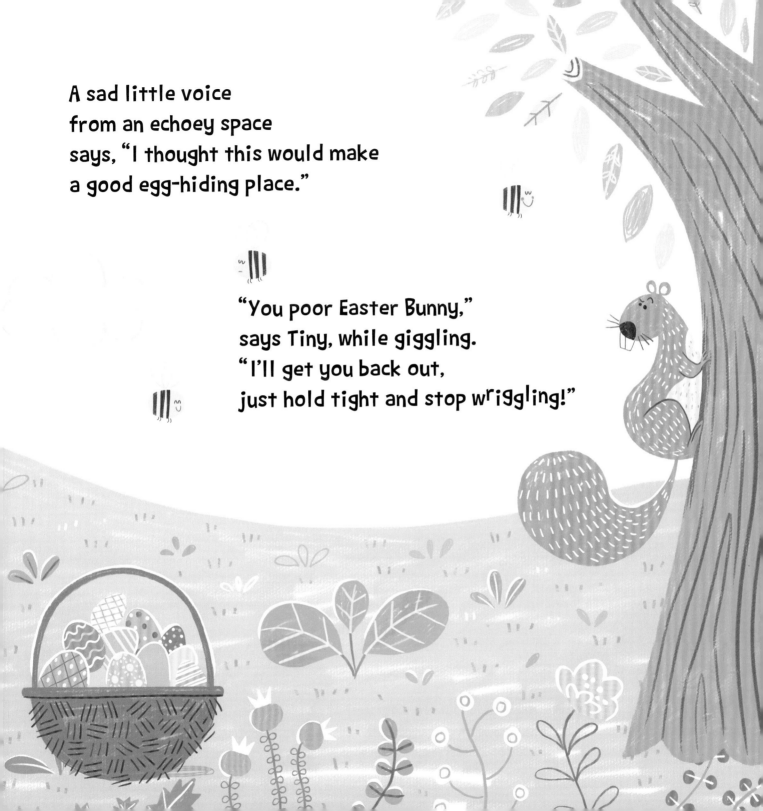

"You poor Easter Bunny,"
says Tiny, while giggling.
"I'll get you back out,
just hold tight and stop wriggling!"

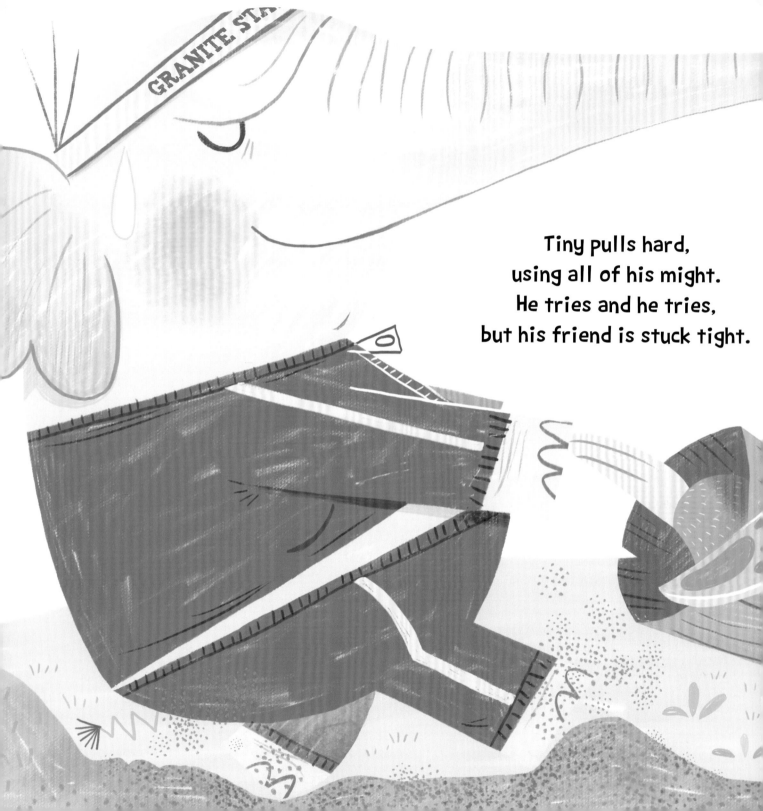

Tiny pulls hard,
using all of his might.
He tries and he tries,
but his friend is stuck tight.

"My eggs," sighs poor Fluff.
"Who'll deliver them now?"
"I'll do it," says Tiny.
Fluff laughs and asks,

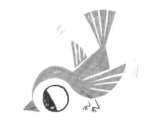

"How?!"

"Don't worry, dear Fluff.
Leave it all up to me.
I watched you last Easter.
How hard can it be?"

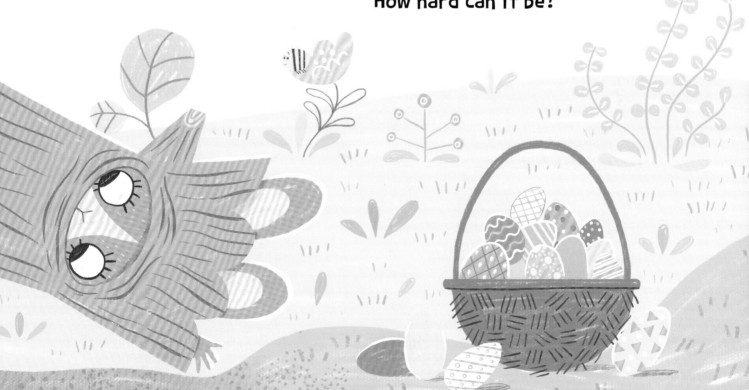

This bunny looks funny... Yes, something is wrong!

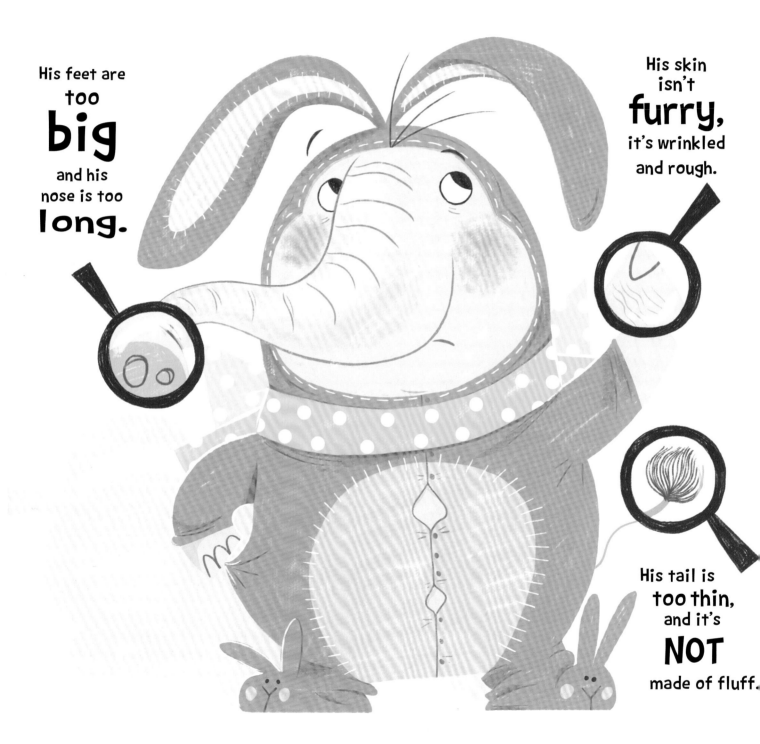

His feet are **too big** and his nose is too **long.**

His skin isn't **furry,** it's wrinkled and rough.

His tail is **too thin,** and it's **NOT** made of fluff.

He's run through **Hanover**
and **Derry** already.
He's all out of puff
and his legs feel unsteady.

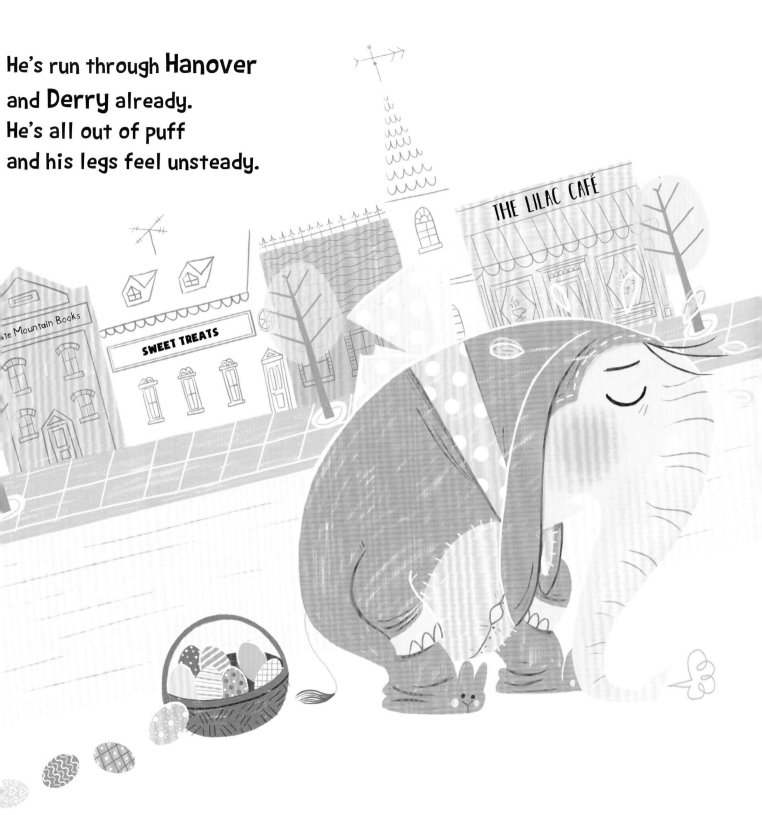

He hops, then he stops,
then he hops a bit more,
then he stops all the hopping...

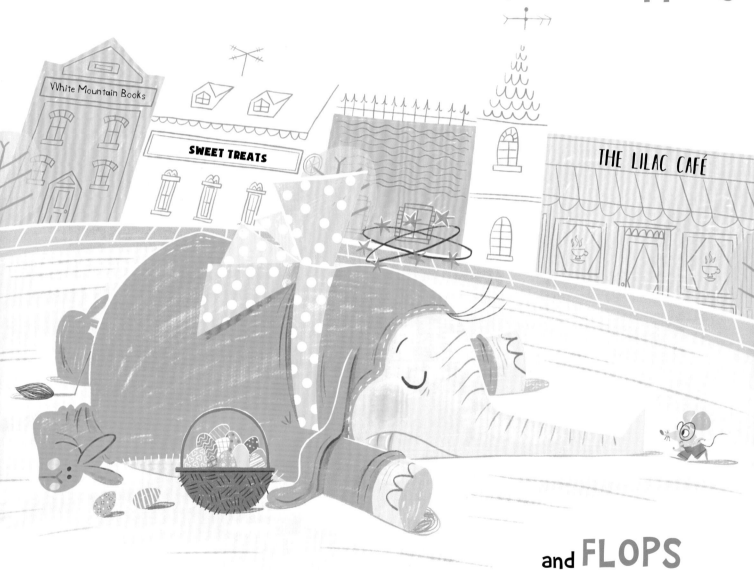

White Mountain Books

SWEET TREATS

THE LILAC CAFÉ

and FLOPS
to the floor!

"Hello," squeaks a mouse
in his fake bunny ear.
"Oh my, how you've grown
since I met you last year.
I'm Marvin, remember?
You're running quite late...
I'll help if you like."
Tiny nods and says,

"Great!"

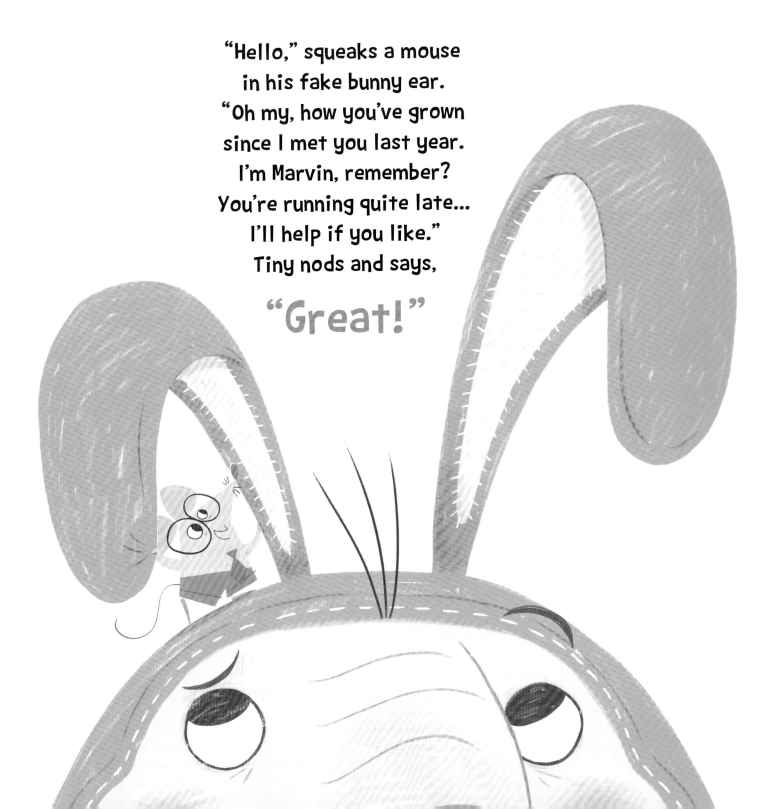

They head down to **Cornish** and rush through the streets, delivering handfuls of chocolatey treats.

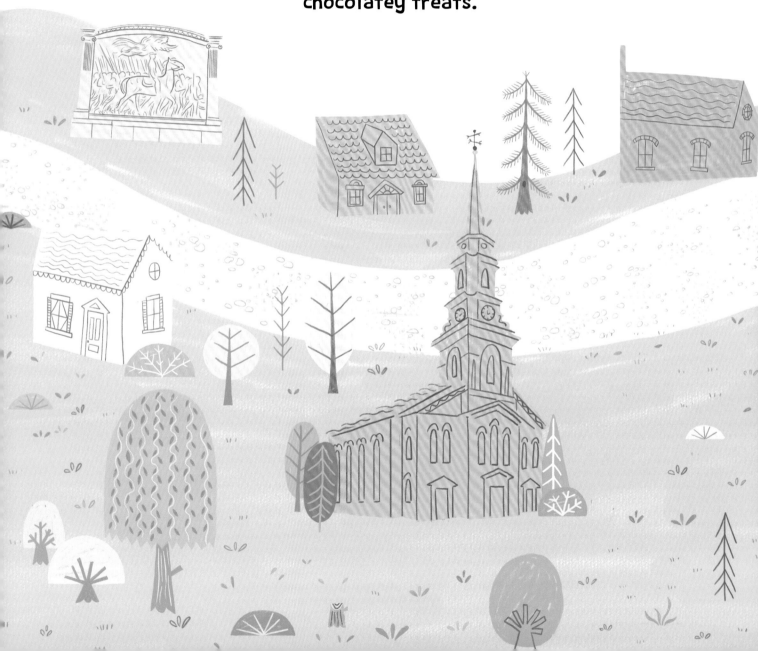

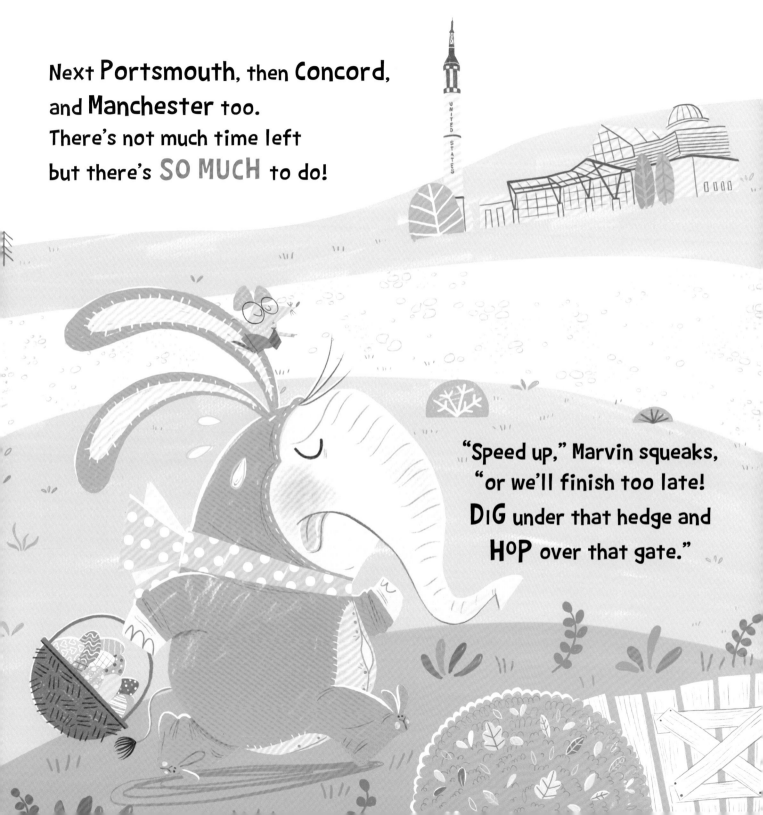

Next **Portsmouth**, then **Concord**,
and **Manchester** too.
There's not much time left
but there's SO MUCH to do!

"Speed up," Marvin squeaks,
"or we'll finish too late!
DiG under that hedge and
HoP over that gate."

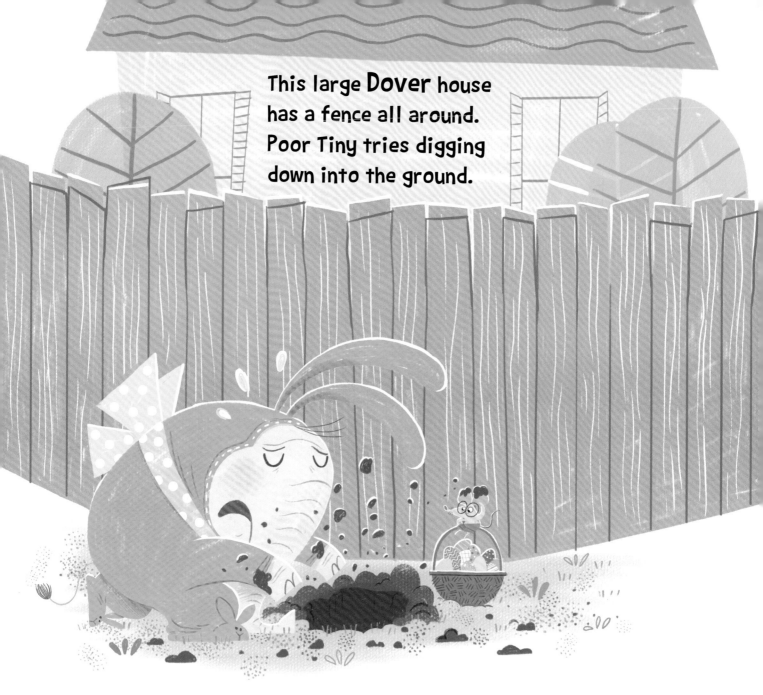

This large **Dover** house
has a fence all around.
Poor Tiny tries digging
down into the ground.

But the hole is too small (or his body's too big).
"How odd," Marvin thinks. "I thought bunnies could dig!"

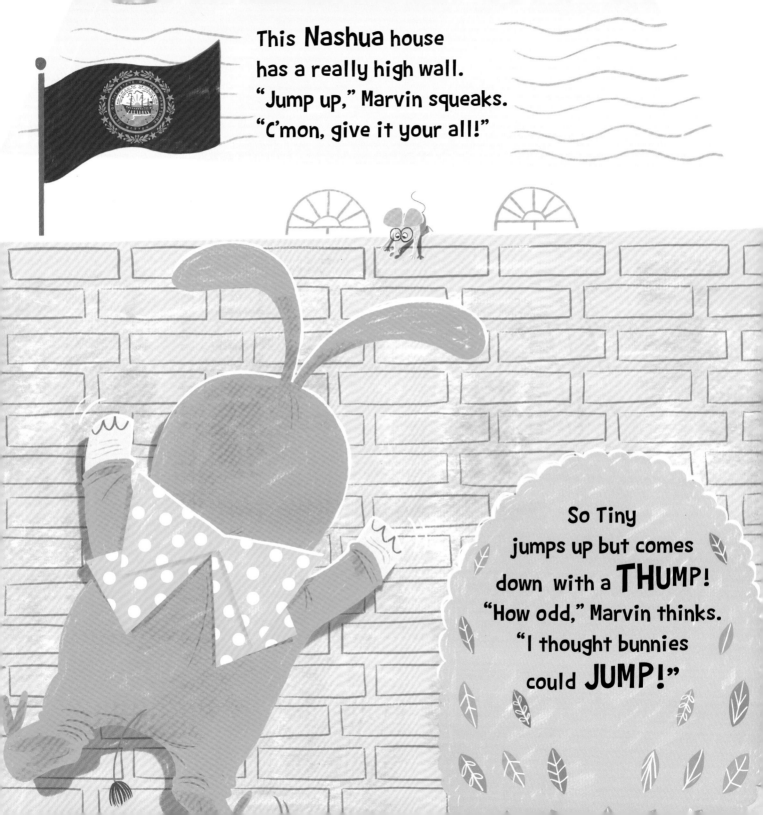

This **Nashua** house has a really high wall. "Jump up," Marvin squeaks. "C'mon, give it your all!"

So Tiny jumps up but comes down with a **THUMP!** "How odd," Marvin thinks. "I thought bunnies could **JUMP!**"

"There's something not right,"
Marvin says. "Let me see..."
He scratches his chin and thinks,
"What can it be?"

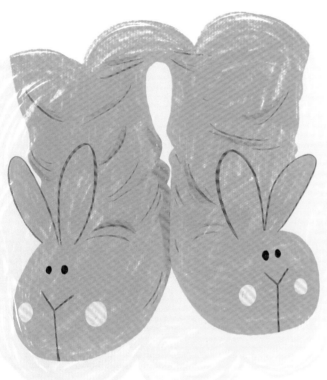

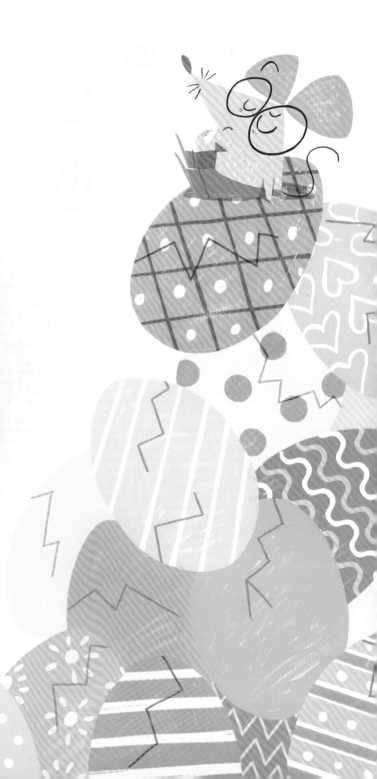

"You're not very fast—
well, just look at those legs!
You're not very careful.
You've cracked half the eggs!"

"You do not have whiskers!
You're no good at hopping!
Those ears look quite fake,
and that's no bunny dropping!"

"Aha! Now I've got it!"
He jumps to his toes.
"No bunny is born with a
trunk for a nose!"

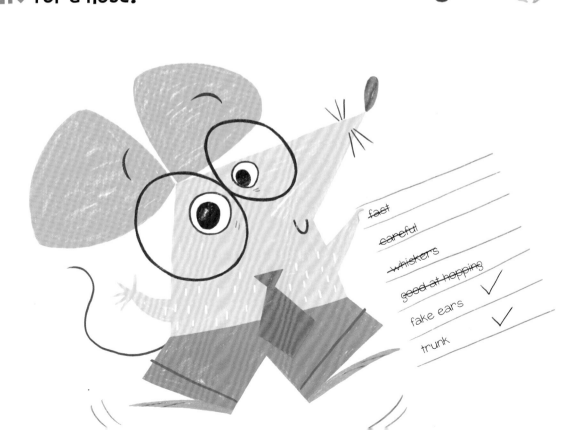

~~fast~~
~~careful~~
~~whiskers~~
~~good at hopping~~ ✓
fake ears ✓
trunk

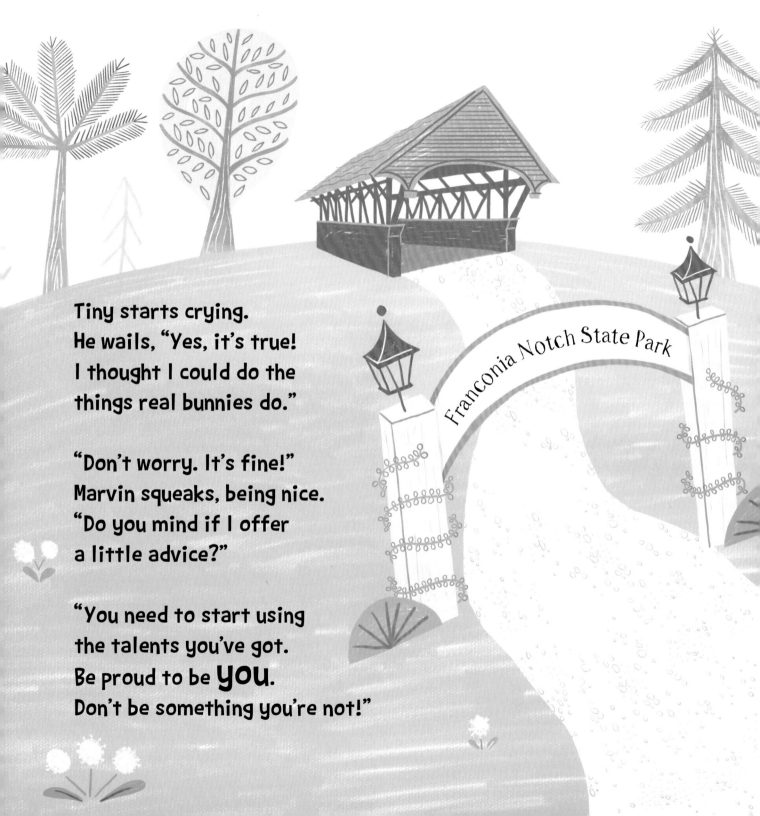

Tiny starts crying.
He wails, "Yes, it's true!
I thought I could do the
things real bunnies do."

"Don't worry. It's fine!"
Marvin squeaks, being nice.
"Do you mind if I offer
a little advice?"

"You need to start using
the talents you've got.
Be proud to be **you**.
Don't be something you're not!"

Franconia Notch State Park

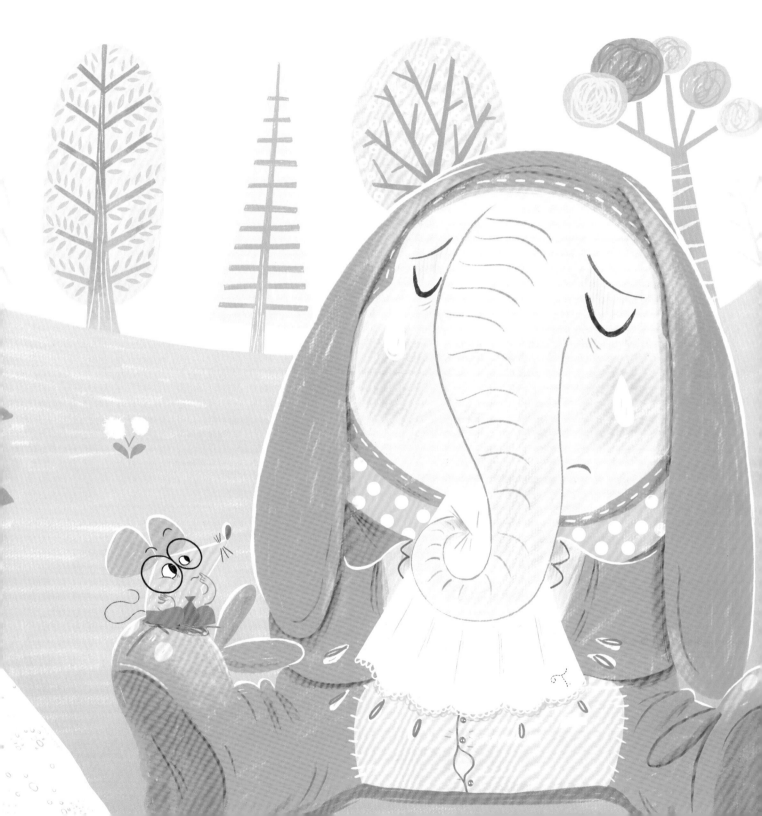

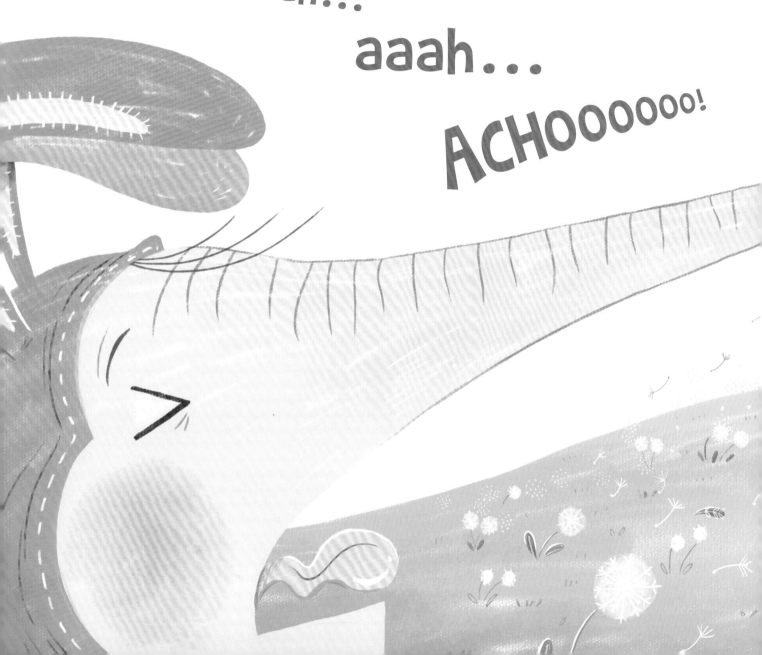

"What talents?" says Tiny.
"What things can I do?"
He blows his big nose
and then aah...

aaah...

ACHOOOOOO!

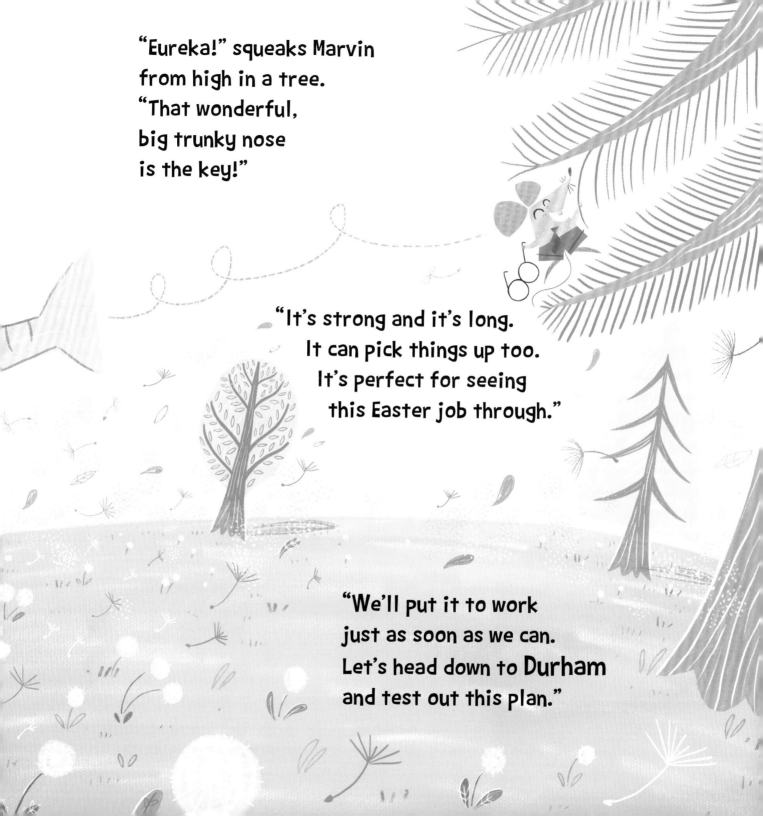

"Eureka!" squeaks Marvin
from high in a tree.
"That wonderful,
big trunky nose
is the key!"

"It's strong and it's long.
It can pick things up too.
It's perfect for seeing
this Easter job through."

"We'll put it to work
just as soon as we can.
Let's head down to Durham
and test out this plan."

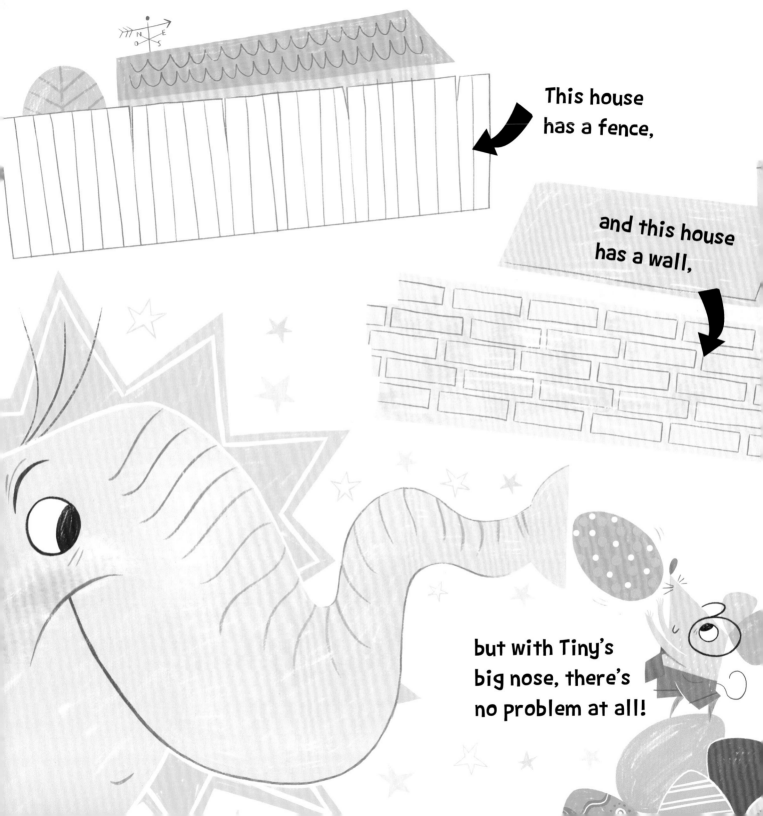

This house has a fence,

and this house has a wall,

but with Tiny's big nose, there's no problem at all!

His long nose lifts up,
reaches over the top,
and he drops an egg down
on the lawn with a

P
l
o
P!

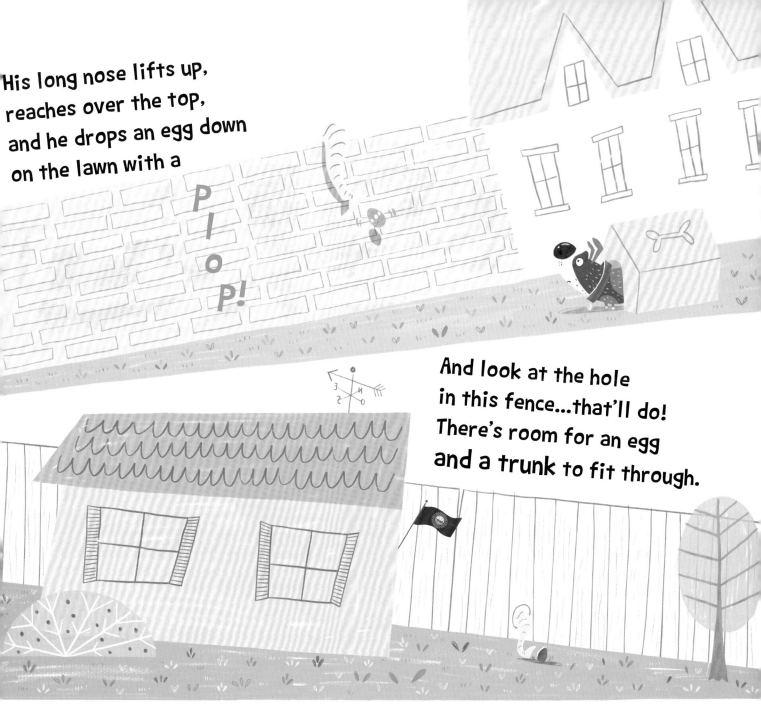

And look at the hole
in this fence...that'll do!
There's room for an egg
and a trunk to fit through.

Now the job seems quite easy. (Well, that's how it goes
when an elephant uses his brains and his nose.)

But daylight is breaking.
The sun starts to rise,
and home after home
stands in front of their eyes.

"I don't think we'll make it,"
squeaks Marvin. "Oh, dear!"
"Hang on," Tiny shouts.
"I've a marvelous idea!"

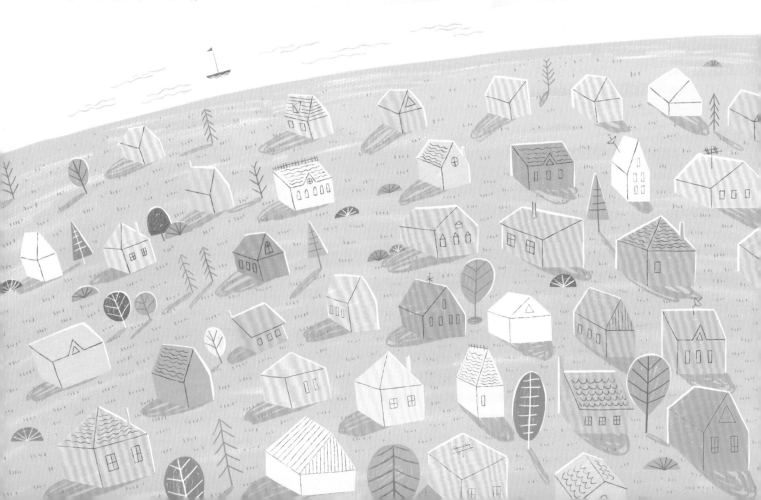

He sucks all the Easter eggs
into his nose,
and when his trunk's full
he takes aim...then he BLOWS!

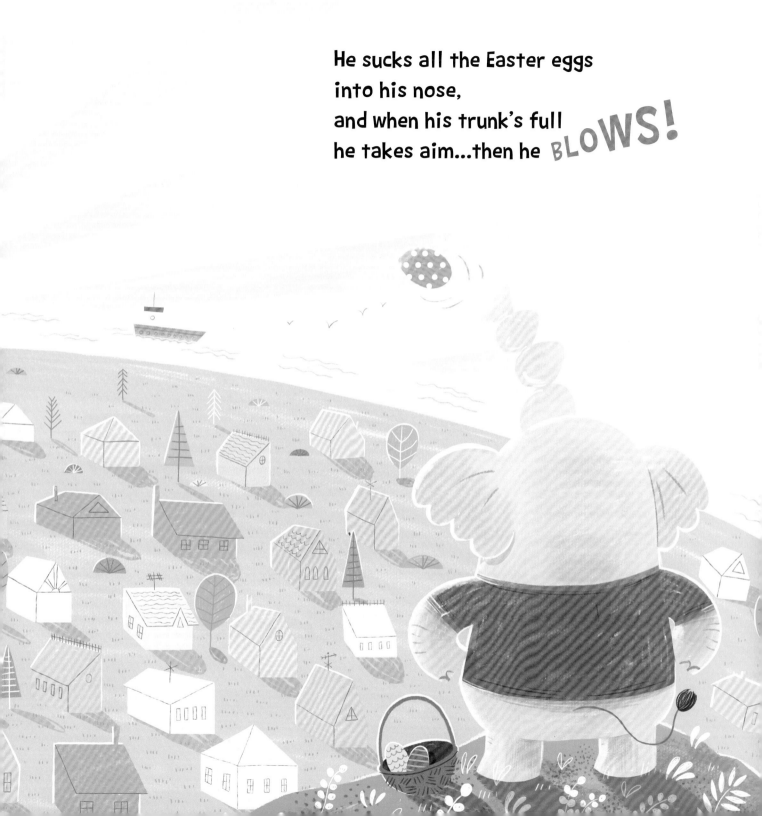

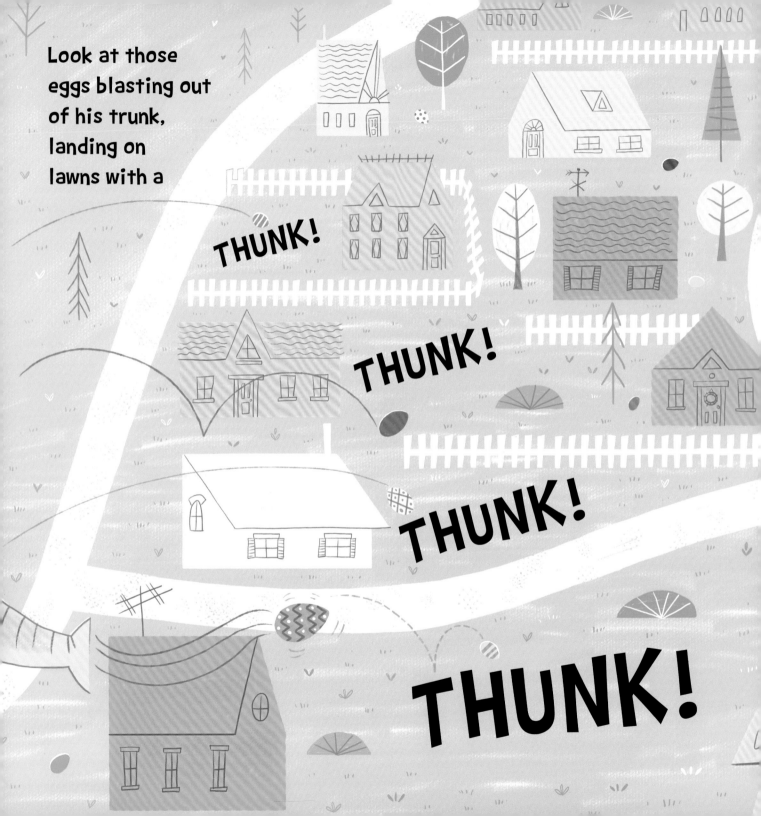

Look at those eggs blasting out of his trunk, landing on lawns with a

THUNK!

THUNK!

THUNK!

THUNK!

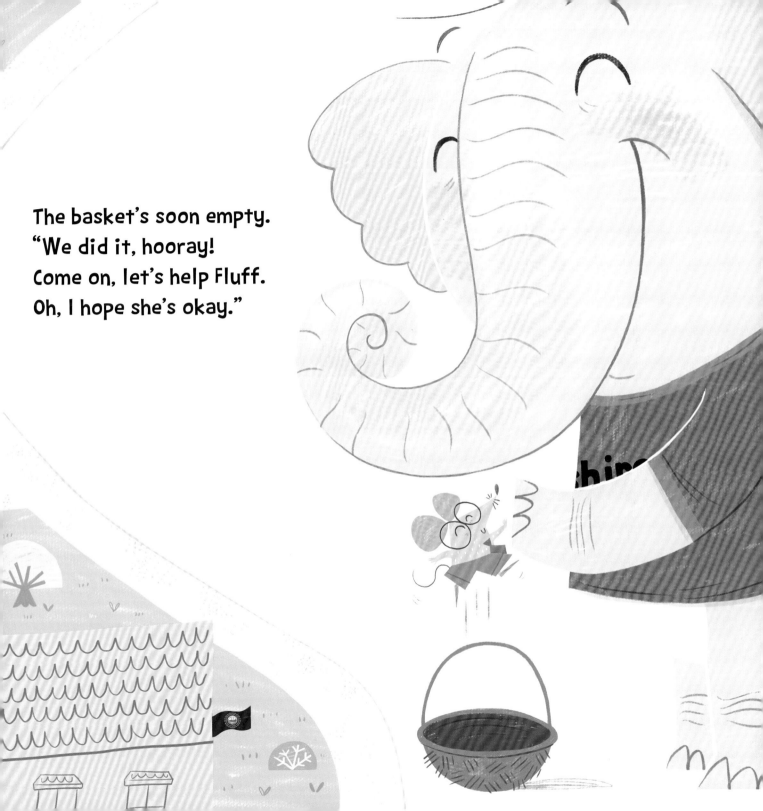

The basket's soon empty.
"We did it, hooray!
Come on, let's help Fluff.
Oh, I hope she's okay."

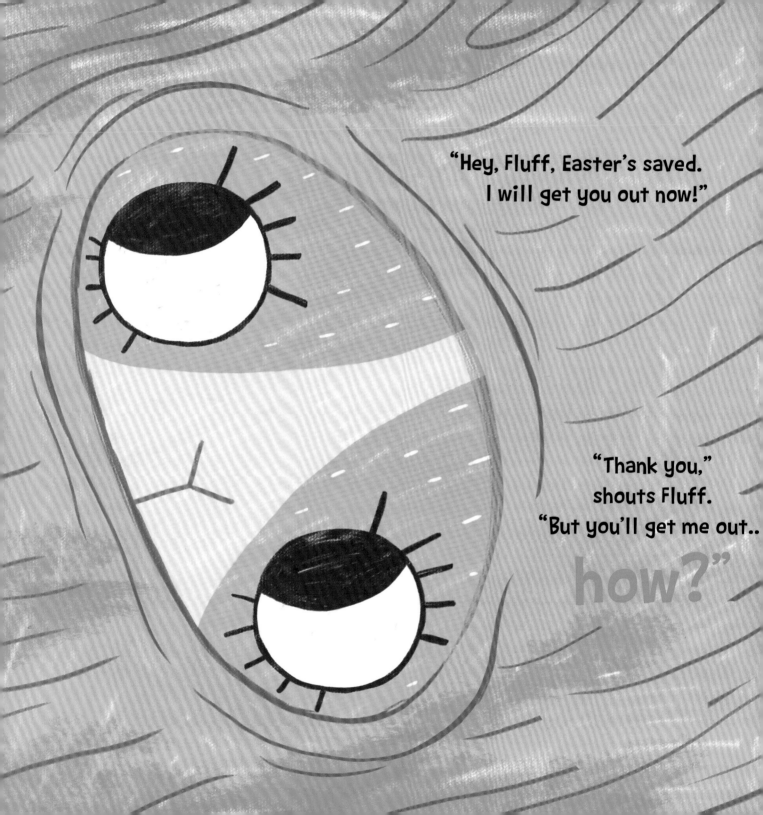

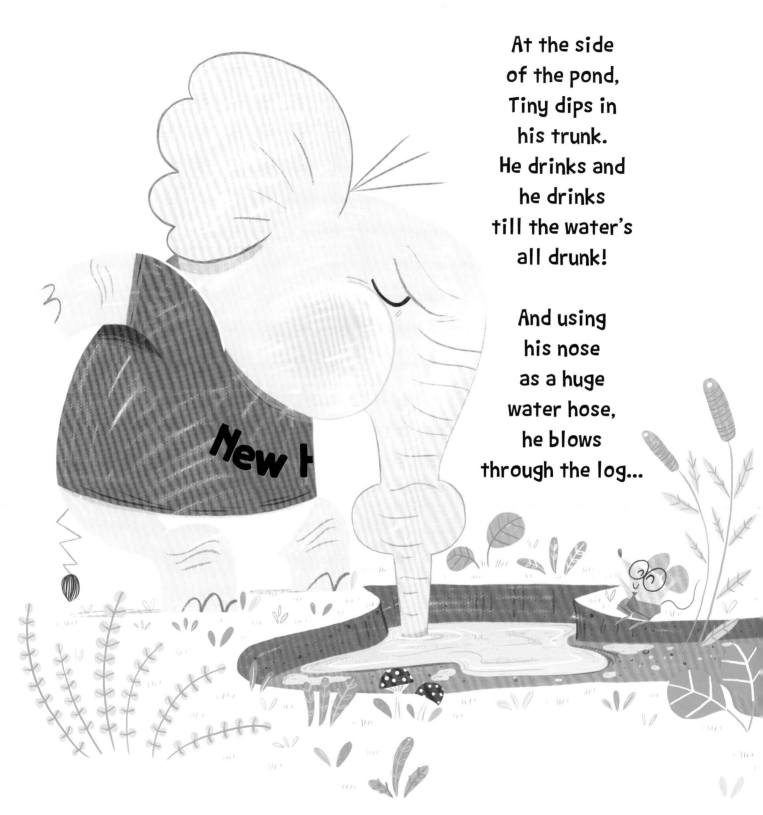

At the side
of the pond,
Tiny dips in
his trunk.
He drinks and
he drinks
till the water's
all drunk!

And using
his nose
as a huge
water hose,
he blows
through the log...

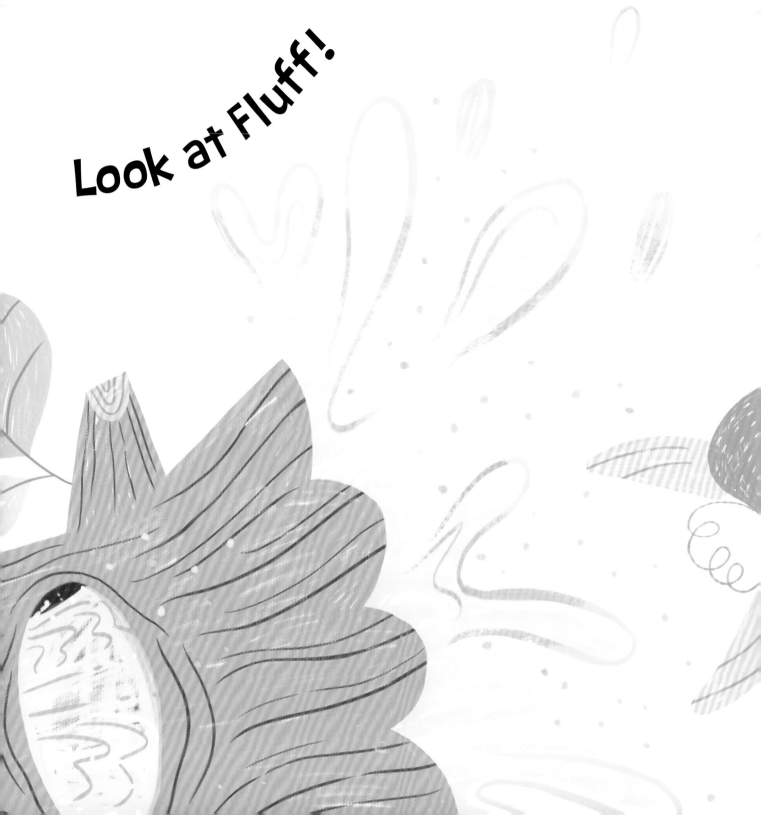

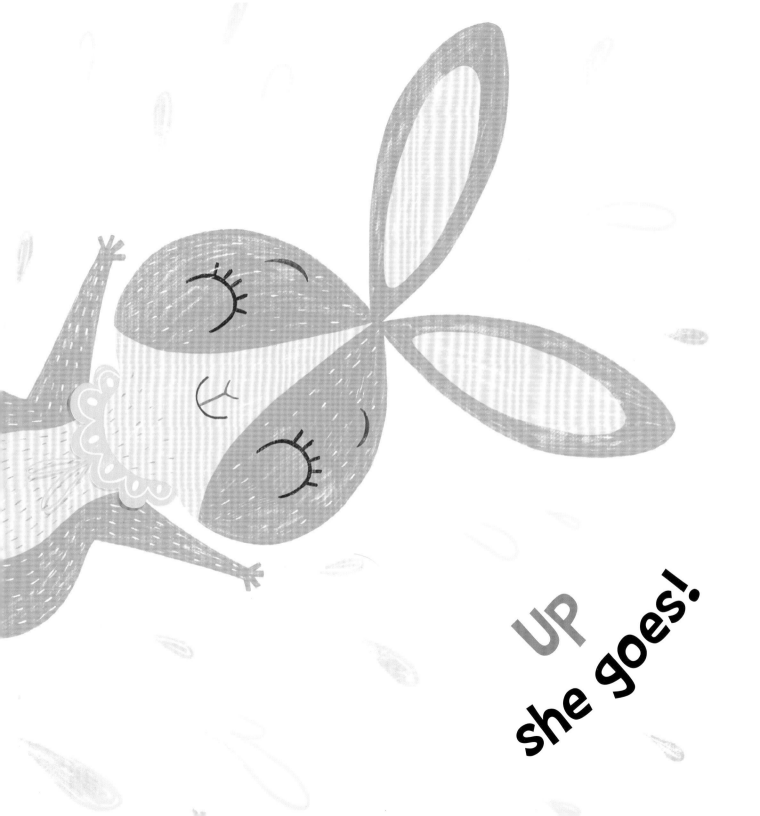

UP
she goes!

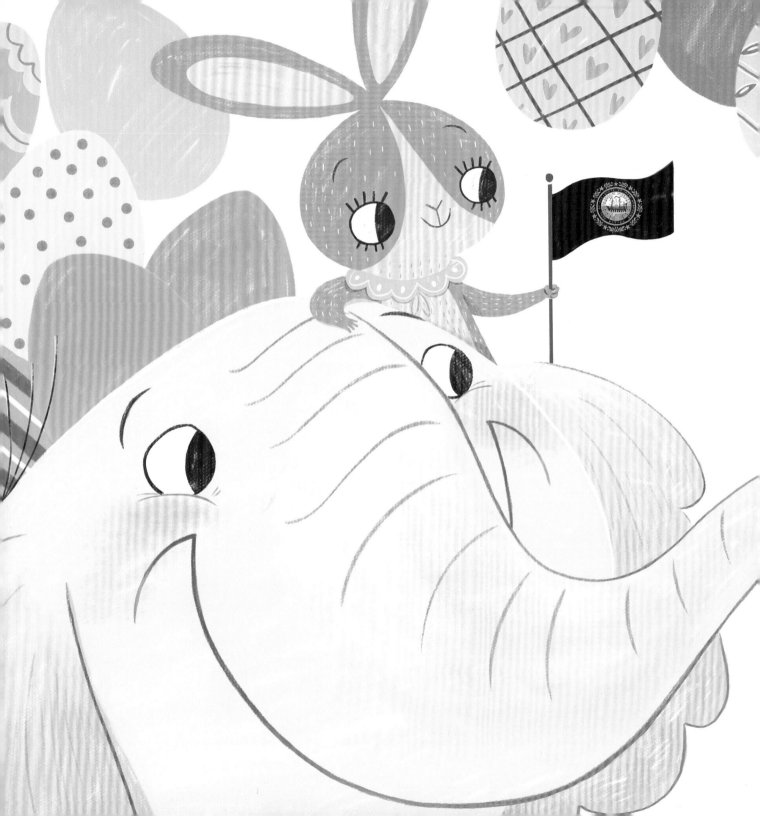

Happy Easter, New Hampshire!

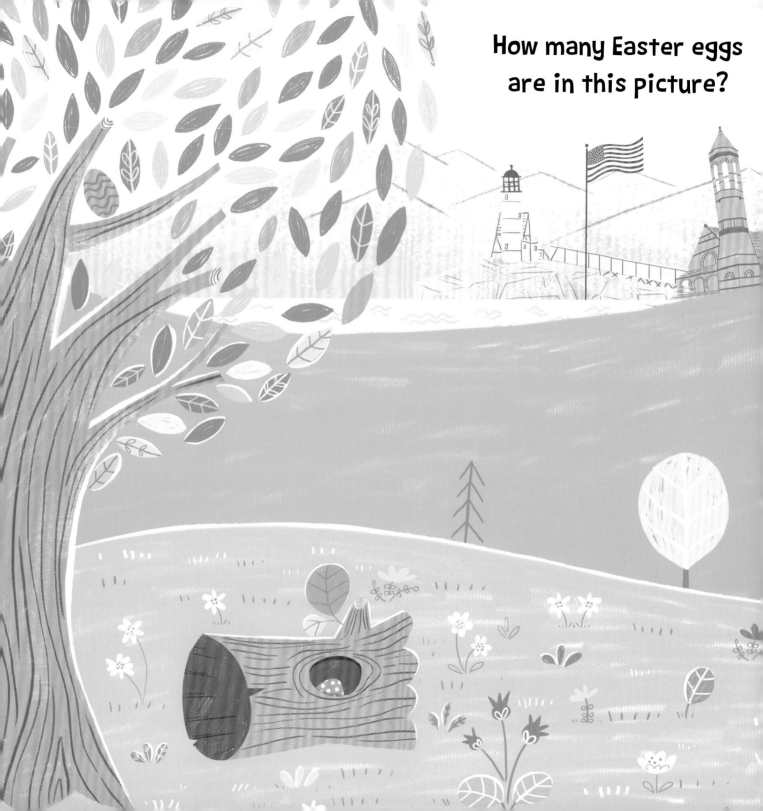

How many Easter eggs
are in this picture?